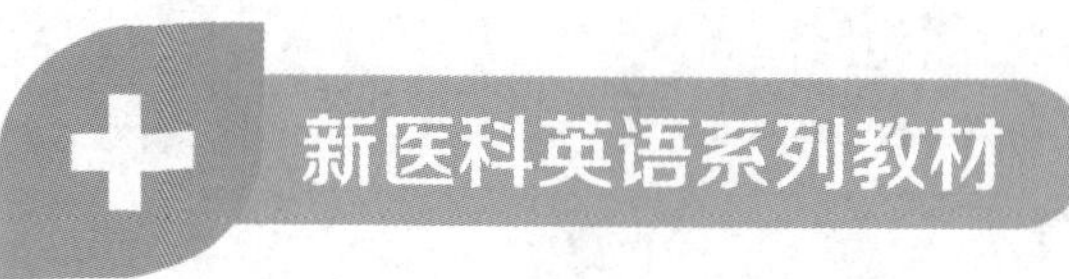

A COURSEBOOK OF MEDICAL ENGLISH WRITING

医学英语写作教程

总主编◎黄立鹤　吴　赟

主　编◎马　文　苏永刚

副主编◎张　晶　孟　晓
刘玉山　丁巧玲
杨　馨　石洪波
孙延宁

编　者◎丁巧玲　刘玉山
马　文　孟　晓
桑　伟　石洪波
苏永刚　孙延宁
田一农　王筱帆
王艳琴　杨　馨
张　丹　张　晶
张　晓

（按姓氏拼音排序）

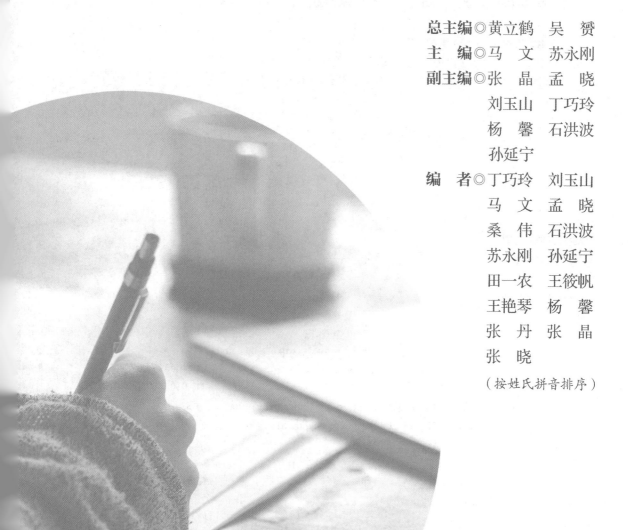

清華大学出版社

北　京

内容简介

本教材以“新医科”为背景，以写作理论为基础，以实用和实践为主线，通过例句和范文，指导学生掌握生物医学语境下一些常见英语文体的内容、要求、特点和写作技巧。本教材共分为两大部分：应用篇（六章）和学术篇（六章）。应用篇涵盖简历、医学信函、医学证明、医用广告、药品说明书、病历等实用文体的写作；学术篇则专注于医学论文标题与摘要、医学研究论文、医学文献综述、病例报告、国际医学会议等专业文体的写作。

图书在版编目（CIP）数据

医学英语写作教程 / 黄立鹤，吴赟总主编；马文等主编.
北京：清华大学出版社，2024.11. --（新医科英语系列教材）.
ISBN 978-7-302-67599-0

Ⅰ. R

中国国家版本馆 CIP 数据核字第 2024P85G87 号

责任编辑：白周兵
封面设计：张伯阳
责任校对：王荣静
责任印制：丛怀宇

出版发行：清华大学出版社
网　　址：https://www.tup.com.cn, https://www.wqxuetang.com
地　　址：北京清华大学学研大厦 A 座　　邮　　编：100084
社 总 机：010-83470000　　邮　　购：010-62786544
投稿与读者服务：010-62776969, c-service@tup.tsinghua.edu.cn
质量反馈：010-62772015, zhiliang@tup.tsinghua.edu.cn
印 装 者：河北盛世彩捷印刷有限公司
经　　销：全国新华书店
开　　本：185mm × 260mm　　印　　张：15.75　　字　　数：316 千字
版　　次：2024 年 12 月第 1 版　　印　　次：2024 年 12 月第 1 次印刷
定　　价：68.00 元

产品编号：097841-01

总　序

中华人民共和国成立以来，特别是改革开放以来，我国健康领域的改革发展取得了显著成就。近 10 年来，健康中国战略全面实施，人民健康得到全方位保障，我国走出了一条中国特色卫生健康事业改革发展之路。医学教育是卫生健康事业发展的重要基石，党的十八大以来，我国把人民健康放在优先发展的战略地位，医学教育蓬勃发展，高素质医学人才脱颖而出。面对实施健康中国战略的新任务、世界医学发展的新要求，我国仍需把医学教育摆在教育和卫生健康事业优先发展的地位。

随着我国持续推进卫生健康国际交流合作、深入参与全球卫生治理，健康医疗领域人员跨国界、跨地区流动已是大势所趋，国际化能力培养在我国医学教育发展中愈加受到重视。《国务院办公厅关于加快医学教育创新发展的指导意见》（国办发〔2020〕34 号）（下称《指导意见》）明确指出，要“培养具有国际视野的高层次拔尖创新医学人才”。2020 年 6 月，教育部临床医学专业认证工作委员会以“无条件通过”的结果正式获得世界医学教育联合会（WFME）医学教育认证机构认定，这标志着我国医学教育标准和认证体系实现国际实质等效，医学教育认证质量得到了国际认可。毫无疑问，提升健康医学领域人才的国际化视野和能力是落实我国“新医科”教育理念的重要方面。

为进一步落实“新医科”教育中的国际化能力培养，提升健康医学专业学生的英语应用能力，我们深度参与了“新医科英语系列教材”的编撰工作，主要承担《医学英语基础教程》《医学英语阅读教程》《医学英语写作教程》《医学人文英语教程》《临床医学英语教程》《中医药英语实用教程》等教材的编写。本套教材围绕与健康医学相关的众多议题，落实加快以疾病治疗为中心向以健康促进为中心的转变，体现“大健康”理念，覆盖基础医学、临床医学、中医药、医学技术、公共卫生、医学人文、医学史、医学哲学等各类题材，涉及健康医学领域的核心范畴、前沿技术、行业标准、历史文化、健康治理等内容。体裁丰富多样，包含说明文、议论文、记叙文、应用文及人物访谈等。教材构思新颖，如把语块教学理念融入基础语言教学，设置真实医学临床实践和研究场景的英语教学，凸显基于医学英语任务的思辨创新能力培养，启发不同健康医学活动背后的跨文化思考，引导学生利用网络信息平台查找专业信息，介绍医工、医理、医文等学科交叉融合的前沿内容等。练习形式有趣、内涵丰富，要求学生对健康医学领域的实际问题进行创新性解决，从而实现英语语言能力和医药卫生专业视野的双向拓展。

全面推进课程思政建设是落实立德树人根本任务的战略举措。《指导意见》明确指出，要“强化医学生职业素养教育，加强医学伦理、科研诚信教育，发挥课程思政作用”，从而培养仁心仁术的医学人才。在编写中，我们始终牢记英语教学的育人功能，融入中国立场、价值伦理、职业素养等内容，潜移默化地引导学生逐步树立良好医德。我们努力平衡语言难度、学术深度、人文温度、历史厚度，在医学科学与语言人文中寻找结合点，力图打造一套既能体现医学人文思想，又兼具国际视野和家国情怀的高水平医学英语教材。

本套教材参照教育部《大学英语教学指南（2020 版）》的课程设置要求，兼顾专门用途英语和通用英语；同时，参考《高等职业教育专科英语课程标准（2021 年版）》，兼顾英语课程结构中的基础模块和拓展模块。因此，本套教材呈现一定的难度进阶，既可以作为应用型本科或高职高专医药卫生类专业的英语教材，也可作为普通高校本科阶段大学英语教学中的医学专门用途英语教材，个别教材甚至可用于英语类专业课堂教学或课后阅读材料使用；同时，它在一定程度上还适合愿意学习国际健康医学相关内容的社会人士，可满足临床医学、护理、药学、医学技术、卫生管理等方向的英语学习需要。

本套教材由同济大学发起，联合北京大学（含医学部）、山东大学、陕西师范大学、扬州大学、黑龙江大学、曲阜师范大学、四川外国语大学、上海中医药大学（及附属龙华医院）、天津中医药大学、广西医科大学、济宁医学院、南京工业职业技术大学、山东医学高等专科学校等高校，邀请医学英语教学、健康话语研究等领域内经验丰富的专家、教师和医生充分研讨、共同编写而成。

同济大学以医学建校，学校始于 1907 年德国医生埃里希 · 宝隆在中德两国政府和社会各界支持下创办的医学堂，走的是一条由医而工、再到综合的发展之路。学校虽于 20 世纪 50 年代在全国高校院系布局调整中将医学院整体迁至武汉，但同济人医学情结至深，历经百年沧桑后，在 21 世纪之初重建医学。近年来，同济医科勇闯创新发展之路，结合世界医学发展前沿、未来趋势及国家需求，加快向国际一流水准迈进。

我们衷心希望本套教材能够配合深化医学教育改革，协助推进“卓越医生教育培养计划2.0”，帮助学习者实现英语语言能力与医药卫生专业视野的双向拓展，培养其在健康医学领域进行国际交流合作的能力，成为我国推进卫生健康国际交流合作、参与全球卫生治理的重要人才。

黄立鹤　吴赟

2023年6月于上海同济园

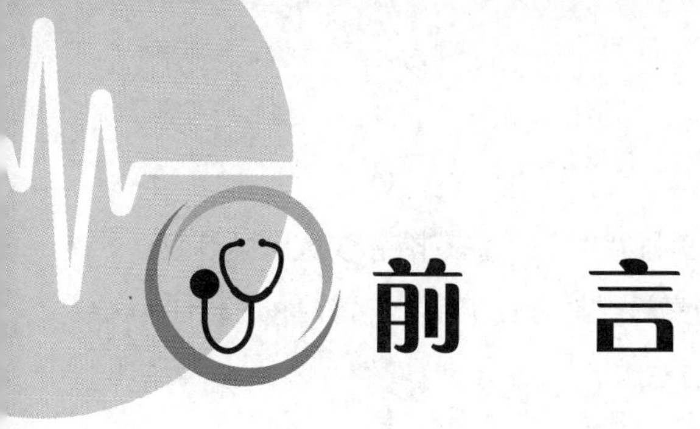

前　言

在当前“新医科”建设教育强国、健康中国战略的宏观背景下，加强研究型、复合型和应用型医学人才培养，全面提高人才培养质量，已成为“新医科”建设的出发点和落脚点。在此背景下，职业教育中的专业英语教育成为英语教学中不可或缺的重要内容之一，其语言教学的基本原则是满足学习者具体的学术和职业方面的需求。但目前，我国大多数本科和高职高专院校的英语写作都侧重于学生英语基本功的训练，而忽视了专门用途英语（English for Specific Purpose）写作的学习和训练。其实，普通英语并不能代替职业英语（English for Occupational Purpose）或专门用途英语。比如在医学范畴内，无论是医学生，还是专业的医疗科研人员，都普遍感到难以应对医学的英文写作，不会用专业规范的英语表达概念；同时，他们也缺乏实用的参考工具，即使有相关教材，它们或缺乏语言学指导，或分类欠科学性，或实用指导性不强。因此，如何将英语教学与医学生的专业培养相结合，如何将英语语言学习融入医学专业学习中，如何将医学英语教学目标更有效地体现在医学英语教材中，就成为医学英语相关工作者所面临的重大挑战。《医学英语写作教程》正是为应对这一新形势和新挑战而编写出版的。

本教材的编写人员都是多年从事针对医学生的英语写作教学、具有丰富教学经验的本科和高职高专院校一线英语教师，教材是他们在详细分析国内医学生写作需求及当前医学英语教学发展需要的前提下编写完成的，旨在帮助医学生在完成普通英语的学习后能尽快适应工作需求，提高他们的英语交流能力和医学英语的专业写作能力。本教材的突出亮点是以写作理论为基础，以实用和实践为主线，通过例句和范文，指导学生熟悉并掌握生物医学语境下一些常见英语文体的内容、要求、特点和写作技巧。

本教材共分为两大部分：应用篇和学术篇，共 12 个章节。应用篇有 6 个章节，内容涵盖简历、医学信函、医学证明、医用广告、药品说明书、病历等实用文体的写作；学术篇的 6 个章节则专注于医学论文标题与摘要、医学研究论文、医学文献综述、病例报告、国际医学会议等专业文体的写作。

本教材提供了大量例句，语料来源既有医学科普读物，也有国际权威医学刊物，语言地道纯正；选用的内容大都是近年来最新的素材，具有真实性、丰富性和时代性。

本教材具有以下特色：

1. 文体实用性强

本教材没有像一般写作教材那样进行简单的写作指导，讲解句子的写作和修改，而是围绕“实用”来进行设计。它侧重于医学生常用的医学实用文体的写作，包括写作的基本要求、文体格式、常用表达、符合业内表达规范的汉英对照具体实例等，非常直观地教学生该怎么去写。本教材针对当今医学英语教学的高要求和医学生的实际写作需求编写而成，具有很强的实用性，可让学生通过学习快速掌握各种文体的写作。

2. 主题突出，融会贯通

本教材强调“医学”和“英语”两个方面，将医学和英语进行有机融合，医学是专业，英语是表达工具。无论是应用篇，还是学术篇，所选例句和范文都紧扣医学相关话题或生物医学论文写作的具体内容。

3. 内容丰富，可读性强

本教材注重突出要点和重点，内容覆盖亦十分广泛。应用篇涵盖医学生和医疗科研人员在学习和生活中可能用到的各种实用文体。学术篇则涉及医学论文写作的各个方面，既有内容讲解，从标题、摘要到最后的讨论，可谓全面覆盖；也有引用方法和参考资料的编排等体例格式介绍；同时，还包含论文写作中时态、语态和惯用语的使用等相关的语法知识。

本教材在编写中参考了《高等职业教育专科英语课程标准（2021 年版）》和《大学英语教学指南（2020 版）》。本教材既适用于高职高专院校的医学英语教学，也适用于其他高校医学本科生、研究生和医学英语爱好者学习。限于编者水平和精力，本教材中的错误或不当之处在所难免，诚恳希望同行和使用者批评指正，不吝赐教，帮助我们在修订或再版时做得更好。

编者于山东大学
2024 年 9 月

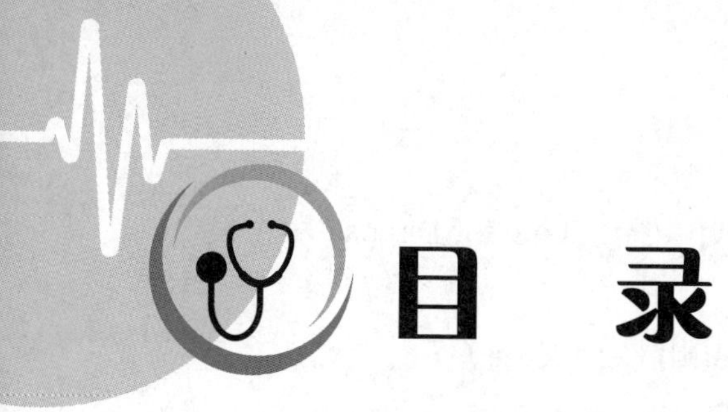

目　录

应用篇

学术篇

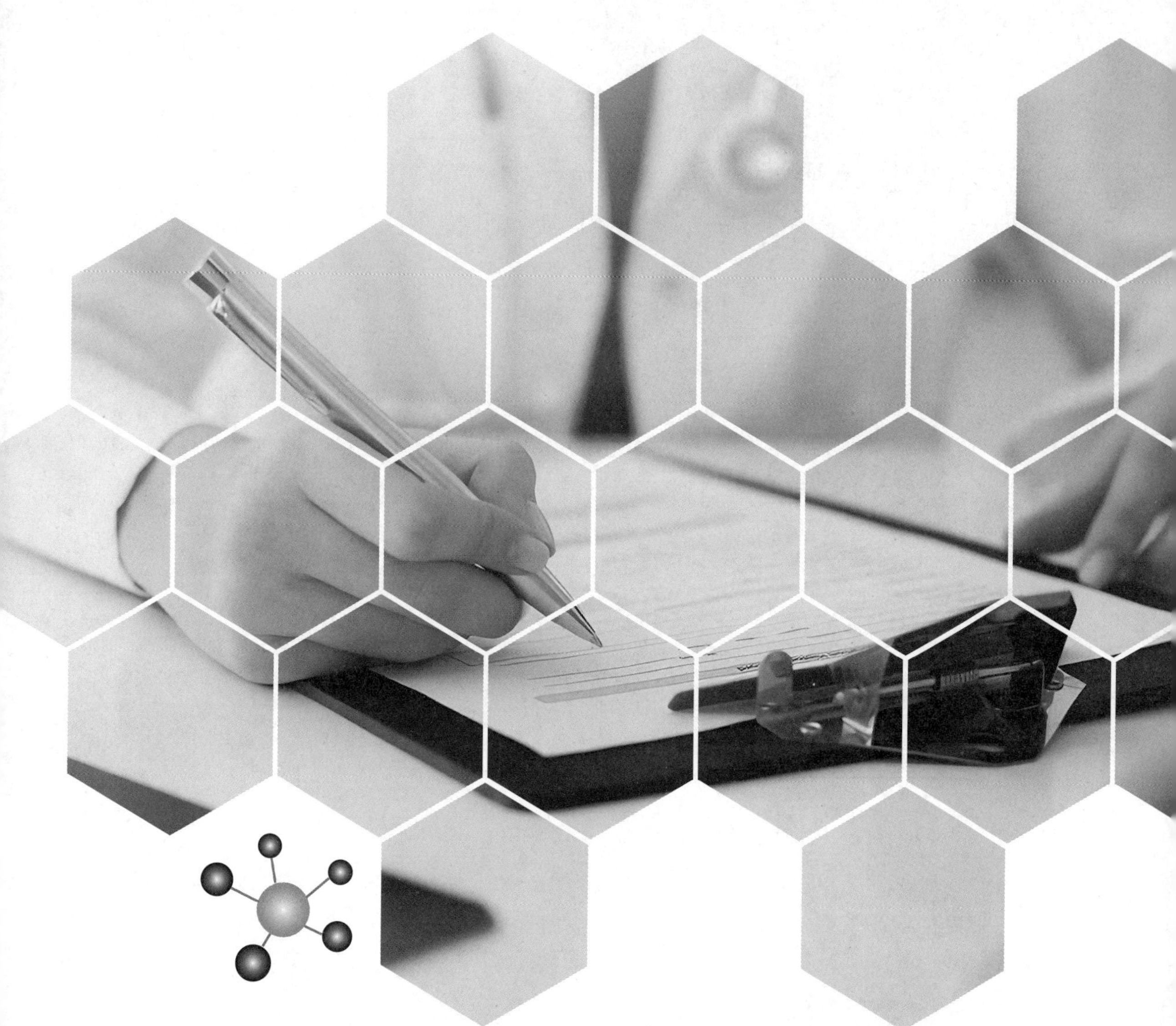

应用篇

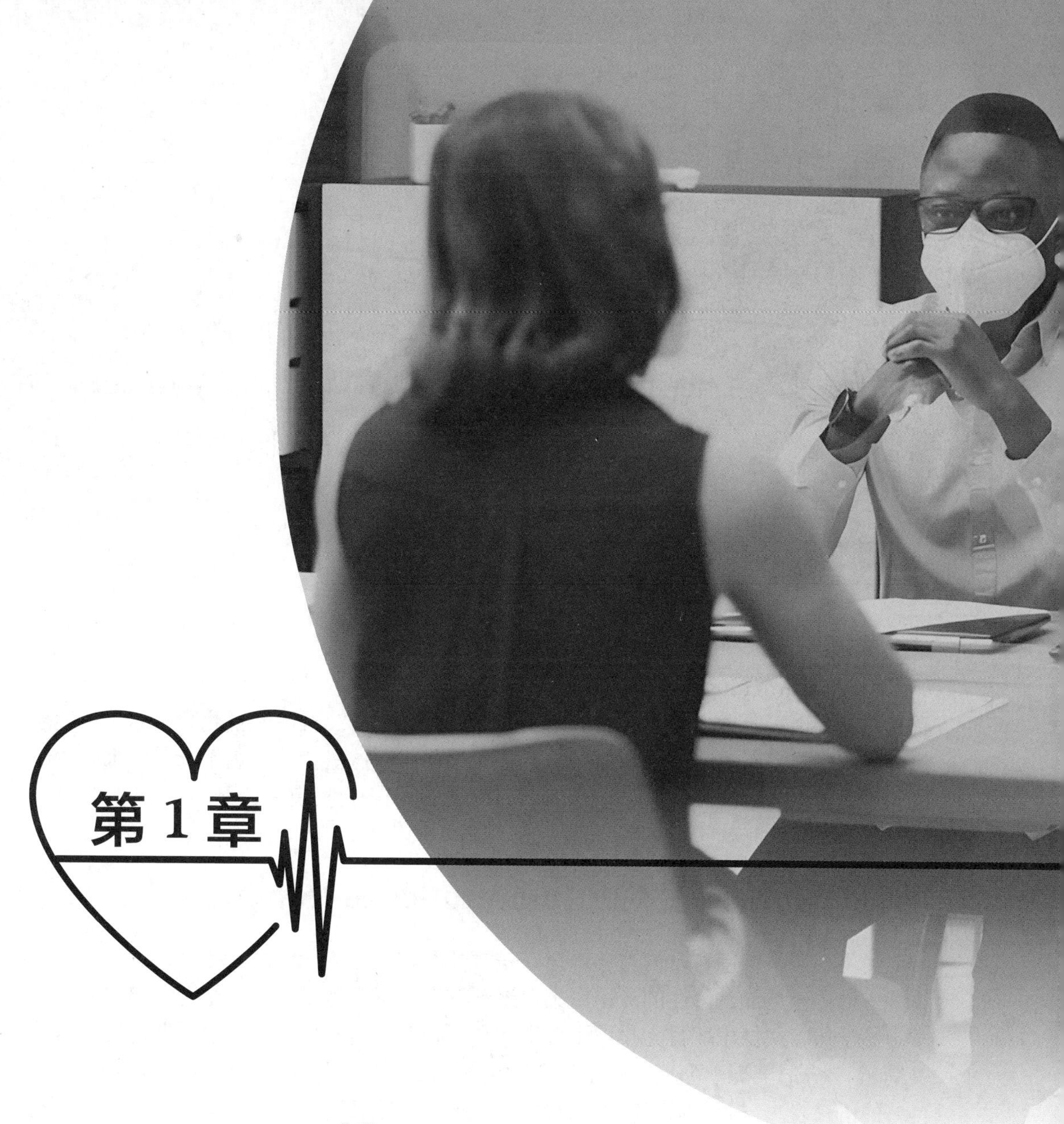

第 1 章

简 历

（Résumé）

Well begun is half done.

好的开端是成功的一半。

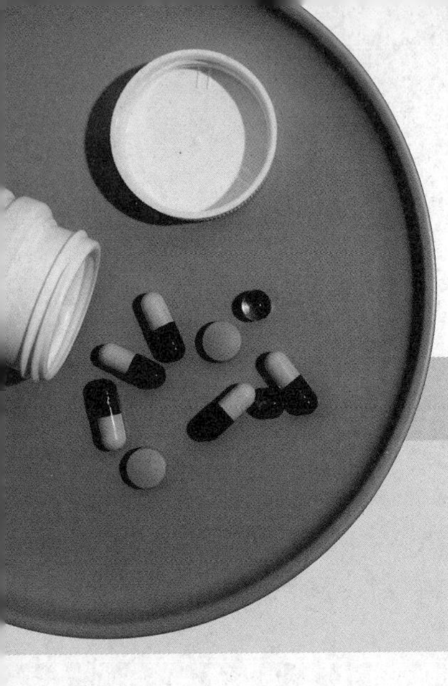

Warm-up

1. How do you understand a curriculum vitae / résumé?
2. Please list items that a résumé should include.

简历（Curriculum Vitae / Résumé）简称 CV，是对个人学历、经历、特长、爱好及其他有关情况所做的简明扼要的书面介绍。简历是有针对性的自我介绍的一种规范化、逻辑化的书面表达。撰写简历通常是为了获得面试机会，常用于求学、求职、申请加入学会、参加学术会议、参加科研合作项目、向刊物投稿等情况。

1.1 简历的重要性（Importance of Résumé）

简历是用来推销自己的首要依据，是打开面试大门的钥匙。近年来，由于大学生毕业人数逐年增加，就业的竞争压力也逐渐增大，越来越多的大学生选择申请国外大学提高学历，或把求职目光投向了外资或合资企业，这些情况下一般需要提交一份英文简历。一份语言规范、得体的英文简历能体现出求学者或求职者具备清晰的思路、良好的语言表达、较强的沟通交际能力，而且能体现出其所具备的专业特长、语言功力、综合文化修养等，因此英文简历的写作是非常重要的。

1.2 简历写作的基本要求（Basic Requirements of Writing Résumé）

简历写作必须目标明确，重点突出，语言简洁明了，版面大方得体，一般最好不超过两张打印纸。简历要实事求是、真诚坦率，不能过于谦虚，也不能捏造事实，且书写要规范，在用词、术语及撰写上都要准确，要用最少的语言传达最多的信息，表述要清楚、无歧义。简历是个人成长经历的缩写，但这并不意味着要把个人的所有经历都铺陈开来，而是应该针对简历的投放目的有重点地加以选择。简历的形式并不是固定的，申请人可以根据个人的具体情况灵活选择格式。一份格式完美、内容翔实、重点突出的简历能带来更多的面试机会。

1.3 简历的分类（Classification of Résumé）

一般来说，根据个人经历的侧重点，简历主要可以分为以学历为主的简历（Education-Based Résumé）、以工作经历为主的简历（Work Experience-Based Résumé）和以职能为主的简历（Position-Based Résumé）等；根据投放目的，简历主要可以分为留学申请简历（Résumé for Studying Abroad）和求职简历（Résumé for Job-Hunting）等。

本章将重点介绍求职简历的基本内容和写法。

1.4 求职简历（Résumé for Job-Hunting）

求职简历包含的主要项目有：

（1）个人信息（Personal Information）;

（2）职业目标（Career Goal）;

（3）教育背景（Education）;

（4）工作经历（Work Experience）;

（5）发表过的文章、著作等（Publications）;

（6）执照与证书（Licenses & Certifications）;

（7）语言能力（Language Skills）;

（8）荣誉与奖励（Honors & Awards）。

具体简历写作中可根据实际情况增减项目。

学生在写求职简历时，由于工作经验少，为了使简历更丰满一些，可以在教育背景一栏写上相关课程，主要突出本专业或跨专业所学特色课程，但是不要为了凑篇幅而把所有课程全部罗列。另外，学生可以将在校期间担任学生干部时组织过的活动细节以及做过的暑期实习等写在工作经历部分。

1.4.1 个人信息（Personal Information / Personal Data）

1. 内容和要求

个人信息即简历撰写人的基本信息，主要包括：姓名（Name），用汉语拼音表示，但中外姓名在姓和名的顺序上是不同的，注意在简历的所有材料中，姓名的写法要始终保持一致；性别（Sex/Gender），大多在姓名前用 Mr. 或 Ms. 以示男女，也有专设 Sex/Gender 一栏，一般填写男（Male）或女（Female）；出生地点与日期（Birth

Place & Date）；婚姻状况（Marital Status）；国籍（Nationality）；地址（Address），应聘外企时务必写上国家名，不能只写城市名；电话号码（Telephone Number），书写时要注意“方便使用者”原则，即尽力为对方创造便利，电话前面须加区号，区号后的括号和号码间加空格，如 (86–10) 8765–4321；电子邮箱（E-mail）是现代重要的个人信息之一，应写在突出位置，单独成行。

2. 示例

PERSONAL INFORMATION

Name: Men Yishuai

Sex: Male

Birth Date & Place: May 20, 1993, in Nanjing, Jiangsu, China

Nationality: Chinese

Marital Status: Single

Address: Department of Thoracic Surgery, Nanjing Cixin Hospital, Nanjing 210000, Jiangsu Province, the People's Republic of China

Telephone Number: (86–25) 8765–4321

Hobbies: Traveling, singing

个人资料

姓名：门一帅

性别：男

出生日期：1993 年 5 月 20 日

出生地点：江苏南京

国籍：中国

婚姻状况：未婚

通信地址：中国江苏省南京慈心医院胸外科，210000

电话：(86–25) 8765–4321

业余爱好：旅游、唱歌

1.4.2 职业目标（Job Objective）

1. 内容和要求

职业目标是指个人希望自己从事并为之而努力的某职业层次及类型组合。叙述目标一般用不定式短语或 -ing 分词短语。

2. 常用表达

To seek / Seeking a position as... 寻求……职位

a private nurse 私人护士

Working in... as... 在……里工作

a clinical specialist 临床专业人员

hospital 医院

stomatology 口腔医学

institute 研究所，协会

3. 示例

Job Objective

To work as a thoracic surgeon in a reputable hospital and utilize my professional skills to improve patients' satisfaction.

职业目标

信誉好的医院胸外科医生的工作，能够利用我的专业技能提高患者满意度。

1.4.3 教育背景（Educational Background）

1. 内容和要求

教育背景是对一个人的学习环境和学习能力的概述。教育背景中需要包含的信息有：学院 / 院系 / 专业 / 学位、成绩、课程，以及其他亮点（个人成绩、取得的成就、在学校担任的职务等）。若申请人是硕士以上学位，不必填写中小学信息；若是通过夜大、专升本获得学士学位，可填本科信息。时间要倒序，最高学历放在最前面。书写学历时，如果正在学习，用 Candidate for 开头比较严谨；如果已经毕业，可以把学历名称放到最前面。关于平均学分绩点（Grade Point Average，GPA）的成绩计算，若非核心课程成绩不高，可用核心课程的 GPA。

2. 常用表达

major 主修

minor 辅修

social practice 社会实践

bachelor 学士

master 硕士

doctor 博士

academic activities 学术活动

in-service training 在职培训

medical faculty 医学院

3. 示例

Education

Sep. 2017–Jul. 2019	Master of Surgery, the Graduate School of Medicine, Wuhan University
Sep. 2012–Jul. 2017	Bachelor of Medicine, Shandong First Medical University

教育背景

2017 年 9 月—2019 年 7 月	武汉大学医学院 外科硕士
2012 年 9 月—2017 年 7 月	山东第一医科大学 医学学士

1.4.4 工作经历（Work Experiences）

1. 内容和要求

工作经历是简历的重中之重，是招聘方非常重视的部分，一般先写目前的工作，再按逆时间顺序写以前的工作经历。工作经历可按年代叙述（Chronologic CV），也可按类别叙述（Functional CV）。工作经历部分常包含以下几个要素：工作时间、工作单位、担任职务或工作内容、主要业绩等。注意：一般一行表述一个工作经历，先写时间，如 2018 至今（2018–present），再写工作单位。工作单位若是新公司、小公司等，可在工作经历后加上长度恰当的单位简介。填写担任的职务或工作内容有助于招聘方了解求职者的发展轨迹。说明主要业绩时，最好给出具体的数字和得到的奖励。若在大学学习期间参加了助教工作，也可写入。简历常用省略句，叙述经历的动词一般使用过去式。

2. 常用表达

be promoted to 被提升为

be proposed as 被提名（推荐）为

achievement 工作成就，业绩

attending physician 主治医师

nurse 护士

behave 表现

conduct 经营，处理

develop 开发

advanced worker 先进工作者

accomplish 完成（任务等）

specific experience 具体经历

3. 示例

Work Experience

Aug. 2019 to present　Qilu Hospital of Shandong University　Thoracic surgeon

<u>工作经历</u>

2019 年 8 月至今　山东大学齐鲁医院　胸外科医师

1.4.5 发表过的文章、著作等（Publications）

1. 内容和要求

求职者需要写出发表过的文章题目、刊登的期刊名称，最好说明级别（国际、国家级、省级等），如果是合作成果，说明自己是第几作者。

2. 示例

Publications

(1) Diagnosis and Treatment of Pulmonary Complications After Thoracic Surgery; *World Latest Medicine Information*; Mar., 2019

(2) Establishment of Thoracic Surgical Difficulty Assessment Scale Based on Delphi Method; *The Medical Forum*; June, 2022

<u>出版物</u>

（1）《胸外科术后肺部并发症诊治分析》,《世界最新医学信息文摘》, 2019 年 3 月

（2）《基于德尔菲法构建胸外科手术难度评价量表》,《医学论坛》, 2022 年 6 月

1.4.6 执照与证书（Licenses & Certifications）

1. 内容和要求

求职者需填写执照和证书的正式名称，不要使用简称或凭印象填写证书名。

2. 示例

Licenses & Certifications

English: Certificate of CET-6

<u>执照与证书</u>

大学英语六级证书

1.4.7 语言能力（Language Skills）

1. 内容和要求

在简历中，语言能力可以是一个公认的语言测试分数，也可以通过一些成绩来证明。例如，雅思、托福、四级考试和六级考试都是公认的英语考试成绩。

2. 常用表达

native speaker of Chinese 母语为汉语的人

fluent in English 英语表达流畅

get a high score 分数高

communicate with 沟通，交流

be proficient in 精通，熟练

I can speak French fluently. 我可以说一口流利的法语。

3. 示例

English Language Skills

Excellent ability of reading professional literature;

Fluent in daily English conversation;

TOEFL Test taken in 2023, score 109.

外语能力

能顺利阅读并正确理解专业的英文文献；

能流利地用英语进行日常对话；

2023 年参加托福考试获得 109 分。

1.4.8 荣誉与奖励（Honors & Awards）

1. 内容和要求

求职者在简历中列出大学与工作期间所获得的与求职目标相关的奖励、荣誉，有助于突出个人的优势与能力。

2. 常用表达

receive 获得

scholarship 奖学金

Excellent Employee 优秀员工奖

Excellent Young Scientist Prize 卓越青年科学家奖

Advanced Medical Worker Prize 先进医务工作者

graduated with honors 获优秀毕业生荣誉

3. 示例

Honors & Awards

Outstanding Graduate Award Shandong University 2022

荣誉与奖励

优秀研究生奖 山东大学 2022 年

Exercises

Exercise I Translate the following into English.

1. 熟练掌握对精神错乱的评估、诊断和治疗。
2. 2022 年大学英语四级考试 595 分。
3. 2021 年获护理学士（武汉大学 HOPE 护理学院）并获得优秀毕业生荣誉。
4. 能熟练地用英语进行读、写、说。
5. 获得优秀实习生奖。

Exercise II Try to write a résumé for job-hunting based on your actual situation.

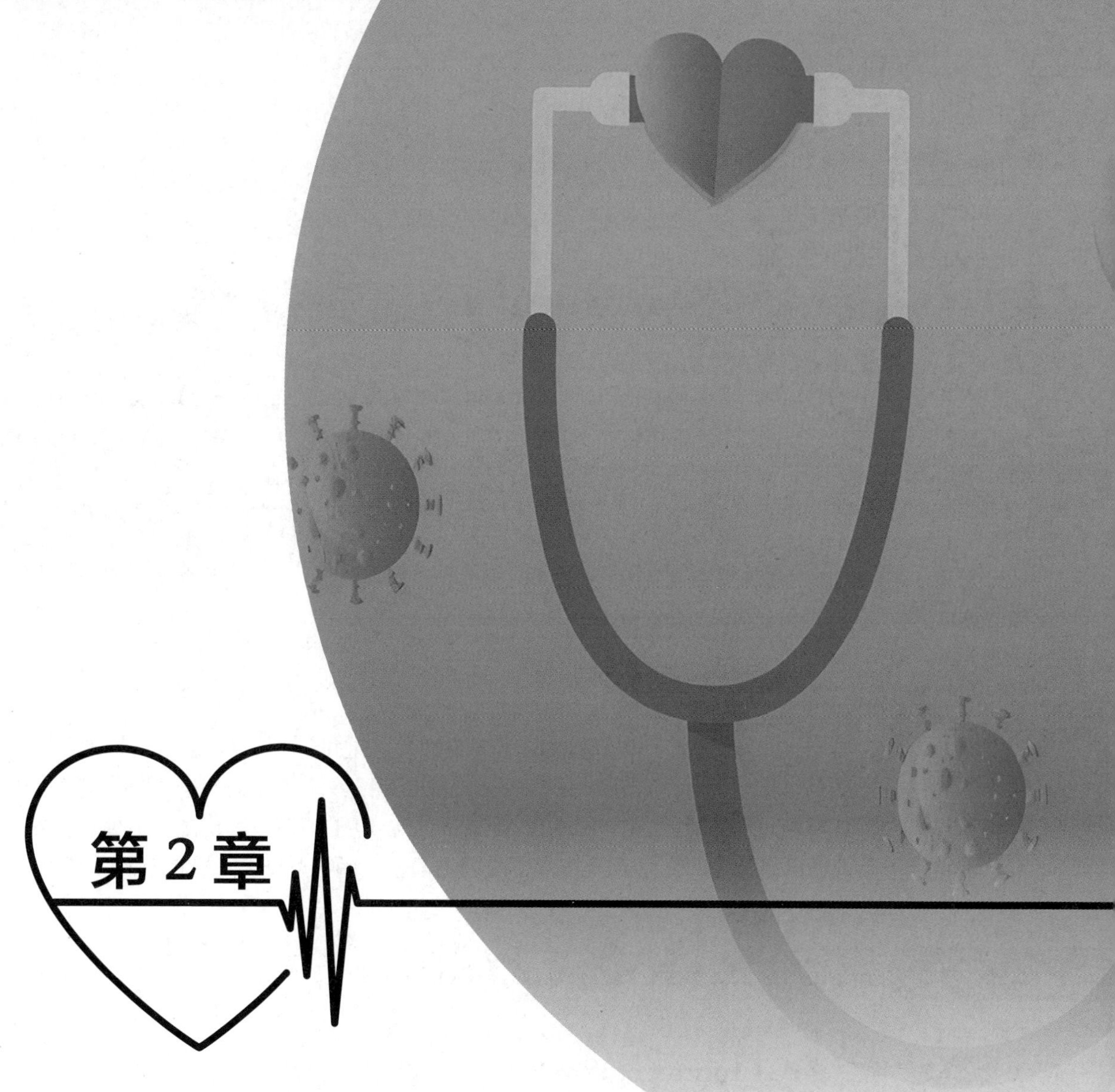

第 2 章

医 学 信 函
（Medical Correspondence）

Hide nothing from the physician.

不要讳疾忌医。

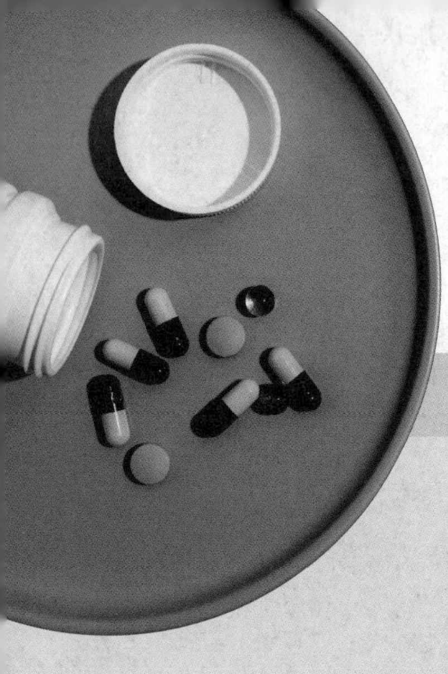

Warm-up

1. What's the difference between medical correspondence and routine correspondence?
2. In what cases is medical correspondence used?

信函（Correspondence）指以套封形式按照姓名、地址递送给特定个人或单位的、缄封的信息载体。医学信函（Medical Correspondence），顾名思义，是与医学有关的信函，内容具有相对严肃性。在如今的信息经济时代，电子邮件以其价廉、方便、快捷的特点备受青睐，但是在医用学术及技术交流等方面，信函仍是非常重要的交往手段。

2.1 书信格式（Format of Letters）

2.1.1 信封格式（Format of Envelope）

英文信封的基本格式如下：

寄信人姓名		邮票
单位		
街道		
省（州）城市		
国别		
	收信人姓名	
	单位	
	街道	
	省（州）城市	
	国别	

（1）寄信人的姓名和地址在信封的左上角，其上边应留两行空白，左边也应留两个字母的空白。

（2）收信人的姓名和地址在信封的中线下方，从中线向左五个字母的宽度处开始。

（3）信封下方左下角可标注：Personal 或 Private（私函）、Confidential（密函）；还可根据需要写 Immediate、Urgent 或 Rush，相当于汉语的“急件”；视需要也可注明 Attention of...，相当于汉语的“请某人拆阅”或“请某人处理”。

（4）信封右上角贴邮票。在邮票下方可打印或书写 AIR MAIL（航空邮件）、REGISTERED MAIL（挂号邮件）或 EXPRESS（快递邮件），均为大写字母。

（5）信封的中间上方可打印 Photo Enclosed（内有照片）、Return Postage Guaranteed（退回免付邮费）。

（6）地址可用缩写词，如 F（Floor，楼）、ST（Street，街道）、RD（Road，路）、AVE（Avenue，林荫道、大路、大道）、DEPT（Department，医院的科室、部门）、HOSP（Hospital，医院）、UNIV（University，大学），但一般用全称。写地址时，英文由小到大，分数行写，最常用齐头式，如：

Northwest University	中华人民共和国
University Road	陕西 西安
Xi'an, Shaanxi	学府大道
the People's Republic of China	西北大学

（7）由被介绍人面交的信，可在信封左上角写：Introducing/Recommending / To introduce，相当于汉语中的“兹介绍某人”。

（8）如系邮寄，但由某单位或某人转交的信，则在收信人姓名下一行加上 c/o 和转交人姓名。c/o 是 (in) care of 的缩写，意为“由……转交”，如：

Professor Henry Acheson
c/o Mr. Abbey L. Mogan
（由艾比 · L. 摩根先生转亨利 · 艾奇逊教授收）

2.1.2 信文格式

英文书信一般由六部分组成：信头（Heading）、信内地址（Inside Address）、称呼（Salutation）、正文（Body of Letter）、结束语（Complimentary Close）、署名（Signature）。有时，书信后还有附件（Enclosure）、附言（Postscript），要视具体情况而定。

（1）信头是指写信人的地址和写信日期，一般位于第一页信纸的右上角，先写地址，再写日期。英文地址的写法是从小到大，先写门牌号、路号，再写区名、市名、省名，最后写国名。日期写在地址下面一行，美式习惯写为月、日、年，年之前用逗号，而英式习惯写为日、月、年。正式函件中，月份应完整地写出来，不缩写。

【例】

Box 408
Peking University
Beijing 100871
the People's Republic of China
June 19, 2023

（2）信内地址：收信人的姓名和地址写在左上方，位置比信头的日期低两三行。英文地址仍是从小到大写出。一般写给比较生疏的朋友的信和公事信件要写出信内地址，而写给至亲好友的信则无须写信内地址。收信人姓名前要写敬称 Mr.、Mrs.、Dr.（可缩写）或 Dear、President、The Honorable（不可缩写）。

【例】

Box 408
Peking University
Beijing 100871
the People's Republic of China
June 19, 2023
} 信头

Professor Edward Ryan } 收信人姓名

Allergy & Clinical Immunology Unit
Massachusetts General Hospital
55 Fruit Street
Boston, Massachusetts 02114
U.S.A.
} 收信人地址

（3）称呼是对收信人的称谓，写在信内地址下空两行顶格写，自成一行，末尾用逗号或者冒号。当给一位熟悉的人写信时可以用 Dear 或 My dear；称呼男士用 Mr.，如 Dear Mr. Smith；称呼已婚女士，在其夫姓前用 Mrs.，如 Dear Mrs. Smith；称呼一对夫妇用 Mr. and Mrs.，如 Dear Mr. and Mrs. Smith；称呼不知其婚否的女子为 Ms.，如 Dear Ms. Mary Low；称呼不知性别的人为 Dear Sir or Madam；如果信件是寄给单位负责人，但不知其姓氏，也可只写头衔，如 Dear supervisor；有些信（如推荐信、介绍信）可分别用于几个收信人，不知道收信人的头衔和姓名时，常用 To whom it may concern，相当于汉语的“致有关人士”。

（4）正文是一封信的主体部分，常在称呼的下一行写出。每行左边的第一个字母都垂直对齐者称齐头式。每段第一行第一个字母缩进 3 ~ 5 个字母空距，其余各行都靠左对齐者称缩进式。两式都可用，但在同一封信里，只用一种格式。

（5）结束语是一种客套语，在正文之后隔一两行的偏右方写出，如 Sincerely yours，后用逗号。

（6）署名的位置一般在结束语的右下方，先手写，再打印出来。如果收信人不认识写信人，可以在署名前用括号标出 Mr.、Miss 或 Ms.。除写给亲友外，签名须写全称，如 David R. Robins 不能写成 D. R. Robins。在名称下面可标注头衔，如：

Sincerely yours,

John Crocker（手写）

John Crocker, M.D., F. R. C. P. (C)

Associate Professor, Pediatrics

（7）附件和附言

附件指附在信内的文件、信函的抄件、支票、汇款单等。如有附件，在信笺末页下方写上 Enclosure，其缩写词为 enc. 或 encl.。若附件为两个或以上，应注明数目，如有 3 个附件，可写为 Enclosures (3) 或 3 encl.。

如果附件重要，还需编号注明，如：

Enclosures：① 3 copies of Annual Report
② 1 copy of translation

写信人要说的内容最好全部写在正文里，不得已才用附言补救。

附言是早期英文信件的常用方式来补充信息，原因很明确：手写信件再改动的话就不好看了。附言（P.S. 或 p.s.）写在签字下 1 ~ 2 行处，写完后再写姓名的首字母。如：

……………………………………………………………………………………

Most sincerely,

(signature)

Lin Yang

P.S. We are especially interested in anesthesia, and would greatly appreciate it if you could send us information on this subject. L.Y.

2.2 医学信函的语言特点和分类（Language Features and Classifications of Medical Correspondence）

医学信函应语气自然，语言简单明了。写信就像说话一样，语气可以正式，但不能僵硬。语言要直截了当，表达要自然流畅，用词要准确。书信交往具有正式

（formal）、真实（real）等特点，是非常重要的交往手段。医学信函有多种分类方法：根据形式，可分为正式和非正式的书信；根据途径，可分为书面书信和电子邮件；根据内容，可分为推荐信（Letter of Recommendation）、邀请信（Letter of Invitation）、感谢信（Letter of Appreciation）、向国外期刊或出版社投稿信（Cover Letter for Contributions）等。

本章将按内容分类进行详细讲解。

2.3 推荐信（Letter of Recommendation）

1. 内容和要求

推荐信是一个人为推荐另一个人去接受某个职位或参与某项工作而写的信件。在特定含义下，它还指本科生或硕士研究生到其他（一般是国外）大学研究生院攻读硕士或博士学位时，请老师所写的推荐信。一般来说，美国的大部分院校要求外籍学生申请入学时提供 2 ~ 3 封推荐信，由教授或工作（学习）单位负责人撰写，直接寄往简章上指定的单位（招生办公室、研究生院或系），不能与入学申请表同信寄去，或者通过系统在网上提交。

不同类别推荐信的侧重点虽不同，但写作时还是有规律可循的。一封推荐信应提供推荐人的身份、推荐人和被推荐人之间的关系、被推荐人的资历和特别技能等，此外还应提供联系方式以供对方了解和确认情况。

下面是推荐信注意事项：

（1）对收信人加以称呼，如 Dear Mr. Dong、Dear Dr. York 等。如不确定收信人是谁，可写 To whom it may concern。

（2）推荐信的第一段应表明推荐人身份及与被推荐人之间的关系，还需表明推荐人写这封推荐信的目的和态度。

（3）推荐信的第二段应该说明被推荐人的个人信息、他 / 她的资历和特别才能，还可以通过具体事例说明为什么为他 / 她写推荐信，让对方更了解被推荐人。

（4）推荐信的第三段应描述被推荐人的能力适合他 / 她所申请的职位。

（5）推荐信的第四段是简短的总结部分，推荐人再次明确自己的态度，如 I highly recommend the person 等。

（6）结尾部分写上推荐人愿意提供更多详细信息，注明推荐人的联系方式并亲笔署名。

2. 常用表达

（1）I have the honor to recommend...

我很荣幸推荐……

（2）I am writing to recommend...
我写信推荐……

（3）I am very glad to recommend / take pleasure in recommending to you..., to be a candidate for the post as...
我很高兴向您推荐……应征……职位。

（4）... worked as a(n)... for... from... to...
……在……至……担任……工作

（5）... is a former student of mine...
……之前是我的学生……

（6）As his supervisor for..., I can state that...
作为他的主管，我认为……

（7）impressive performance
令人称赞的表现

（8）be enthusiastic about...
热衷于……

（9）reliable/dependable
可靠的，可信赖的

（10）ability to work independently
独立工作的能力

（11）a brilliant/talented student
有天赋的学生

（12）... has shown...
……表现出……

（13）be applying for admission to...
申请进入……

3. 示例

Dear Sirs,

Mei Qiming is a graduate student of Xiangya School of Medicine at Central South University pursuing a Master's Degree in Biochemistry. I am his advisor and have known him well.

He is distinguished by his diligence, integrity, thorough-going spirit in research and willingness to help others.

He ranked the fifth among the 40 students in his undergraduate class and got the second highest mark last year among candidates for the Master's Degree in Biochemistry in our department. He received good comments from Professor Jennie Fairman of Wisconsin State University, who gave lectures at our university last term.

Mei Qiming has great potential for research, having an extensive command of basic medical courses. He now intends to prepare himself for the study of the biochemical functions of selenium and its relation to some vitamins. So I encouraged him to study at your university, where several outstanding biochemists are working.

I shall consider it a great favor if you would be kind enough to admit him and give him the scholarship he is applying for.

I earnestly hope that your decision in his case will be a favorable one.

Sincerely yours,

Ma Yurong

Professor of Biochemistry

尊敬的先生们：

梅启明是中南大学湘雅医学院的研究生，作为他的导师，我很了解他。

他的特点是勤奋、正直，研究认真，乐于助人。

他读本科时，在40人的班上名列第五。去年，考生化硕士研究生，在30名考生中，他的分数高居第二。上学期，威斯康星大学珍妮·菲尔曼教授来我校讲课，对他的评价很好。

梅启明在研究工作中有很大潜力，对医学基础课掌握的范围较广。他现在准备研究硒的生化作用及其与某些维生素的关系。因此，我鼓励他到贵校学习，因为贵校有许多杰出的生化学家。

如果贵校录取他，并同意给他所申请的奖学金，我将十分感谢。

我真诚地希望你们的决定对他有利。

诚挚的，

生化教授

马玉荣

2.4 邀请信（Letter of Invitation）

1. 内容和要求

邀请信一般适用于比较正式的场合，如会议、学术活动、开业典礼、展会等。邀请信通常包含以下内容：邀请人、邀请对象、邀请对方的目的、活动举办的时间和地点、期待或感激。

2. 常用表达

（1）Any topic you prefer would be welcome.
任何题目均可。

（2）We should be very grateful If you could...
若您……我们将不胜感激……

（3）I hereby invite you to join our hospital and wish you the best for your new role here.
我谨邀请您加入我们医院，祝您在新的工作中一切顺利。

（4）We are looking forward to meeting you soon.
我们盼望很快与您见面。

（5）We sincerely hope that you could accept our invitation.
我们诚挚地希望您能接受邀请。

（6）With warm personal regards.
致以热情的问候。

（7）Should you or one of your colleagues wish to visit the interesting event, perhaps you will be kind enough to let me know and I will arrange to send you as many tickets as you want.
如果您或您的同事想出席这个有趣的活动，望告知，以便遵嘱安排送票事宜。

（8）If you can come, please let us know as soon as possible, and we will have to prepare the final program soon.
若您能来参加，请尽早告知，因为我们很快要准备最终计划。

3. 示例

Dear Mr. Rodger,

We should be very grateful if you could give a talk to our College of Stomatology at eight o’clock, Friday morning, September 23. As you know, the department is interested in your latest research on Caries Etiology. The audience are all the dentists in our hospital and the interns in our department.

Looking forward to your acceptance.

Cordially,

(signature)

XXX

September 10, 2022

尊敬的罗杰先生，

若您能于 9 月 23 日星期五早上八点来我口腔医院作报告，我们将不胜感激。如您所知，本科室对您最近有关龋齿病因学的研究很感兴趣。听众是我院所有牙科医生和在我科室的实习生。

热切盼望您能接受邀请。

诚挚的，

（签名）

XXX

2022 年 9 月 10 日

2.5 感谢信（Letter of Appreciation）

1. 内容和要求

感谢信是用来表达感谢之情的信件，如感谢提供面试机会、感谢提供工作机会、感谢提供实习机会等。感谢信的用语要求是精炼、简洁，遣词造句要把握好度，不可过分雕饰，否则会给人一种不真实、虚伪的感觉。

2. 常用表达

（1）Thank you for taking the time to interview me on Tuesday for the sales manager position with Williams Black.

感谢您和威廉姆斯 · 布莱克先生在周二对我进行销售经理职位的面试。

（2）I am definitely interested in this position with your company.

我对贵公司的该职位非常感兴趣。

（3）Please do not hesitate to contact me if you need additional information.

若需要了解其他信息，请随时与我联系。

（4）I thank you for this excellent/invaluable opportunity.

感谢您给了我这个宝贵的机会。

3. 示例

Dear Mr. Johnson,

This summer's internship with your company was a truly incredible experience, and I thank you for this excellent opportunity. The internship has allowed me to learn, expand my skills, and revise my future career goals. I know the experience that you have provided will affect me for the years to come.

Thank you again for this invaluable opportunity. I look forward to staying in touch with you and your staff members.

Best regards,

XXX

August 20, 2022

尊敬的约翰逊先生：

暑假在贵公司的实习经历真是不可思议，非常感谢您给了我这次机会。它使我学到了知识，扩展了自身技能，修订了未来的职业目标。您所提供的此次经历将会影响我的未来。

再次感谢这个非常宝贵的机会。期望能和您及您的工作人员保持联系。

最好的祝愿，

XXX

2022 年 8 月 20 日

2.6 向国外期刊或出版社投稿信（Cover Letter for Contributions）

1. 内容和要求

向国外期刊或出版社投稿，最重要的自然是稿件的质量或价值，但也要做好一些准备工作。除了选择期刊，我们还要对拟投稿的期刊有充分了解。寄稿时，一般附信一封。内容主要是说明投稿目的，表明是初稿还是修改稿，写清文章题目和作者姓名，介绍稿件特点，并提合理要求。此外，我们还应声明该文章此前未在其他刊物发表，也未计划向别处投稿，而且要注意行文简洁、观点明确、措辞礼貌委婉。许多期刊都刊有编辑姓名，写信尽量避免用 Dear Sir 作收件人称呼。

2. 常用表达

（1）I am sending a manuscript entitled... by... which I should like to submit for possible publication in the journal of...

本人提交由……撰写的题为……的稿件，不知是否有可能在贵刊……发表。

（2）We believe that… would be of interest to the journal's readers.

我们相信……将会引起该期刊读者的兴趣。

（3）It is more than… since I submitted my manuscript (No. …) for possible publication in your journal.

本人提交拙作（号码……）于贵刊待发表已超过……

（4）I should appreciate your letting me know what you have decided as soon as possible.

若能尽快告知，将感激之至。

3. 示例

Dear Dr. Nixon,

The enclosed manuscript entitled "Appendix Mass in the Very Young Children" is written by Men Yishuai and Su Jie. It is submitted for consideration of its suitability for publication in your journal.

The final manuscript has been seen and approved by all the authors and they have taken their due care to ensure the integrity and the scientific value of the work. Our manuscript has not been previously sent elsewhere and is being considered only by *The Journal of the American Medical Association.*

It is highly appreciated for your consideration of our manuscript for publication in your journal.

Sincerely yours,

XXX

March 17, 2022

尊敬的尼克松博士：

随函寄去手稿《婴幼儿的阑尾包块》，作者为门一帅和苏杰。请考虑是否适合在贵刊发表。

本文定稿时，经全体作者审阅并认可。作者们保证稿件的真实性及科学价值。本稿未作他投，只投给贵刊《美国医学会杂志》。

如蒙贵刊发表，不胜感激。

诚挚的，

XXX

2022 年 3 月 17 日

Exercises

Exercise I　Translate the following into English.

1. 很荣幸接受您的邀请参加此次国际会议。
2. 我热切盼望能够在十月份的会议上见到您。
3. 过去三年间，门一帅是我院的药剂师，特此证明。
4. 我们感谢您考虑我们的文稿。
5. 湖南省省立医院口腔科邀请您作为特邀发言人参加年度会议。

Exercise II　Translate the following into Chinese.

1. You are an internationally acclaimed scholar and educator. Your participation will be among the highlights of the conference.
2. Thank you for your letter of May 20 agreeing to undertake the publication of the work I had sent you. Please advise me when you think it will be published.
3. If the period is not convenient, please inform me as soon as possible of the dates on which you would prefer to see me so that I can make the necessary alternative arrangements based on your suggested dates.

Exercise III　Translate the following letter of recommendation into English.

兹证明（持函人）门一帅先生在我医院工作三年。他是非常称职的会计，细心且计算准确。他字写得好，其他工作也完成得很好。我作为他的直接领导，可以证明他非常勤奋，与同事关系融洽。他现在想找一份责任更大、待遇更好的工作，他有足够的能力。我很遗憾不能挽留他，但是有信心推荐他去贵单位工作。

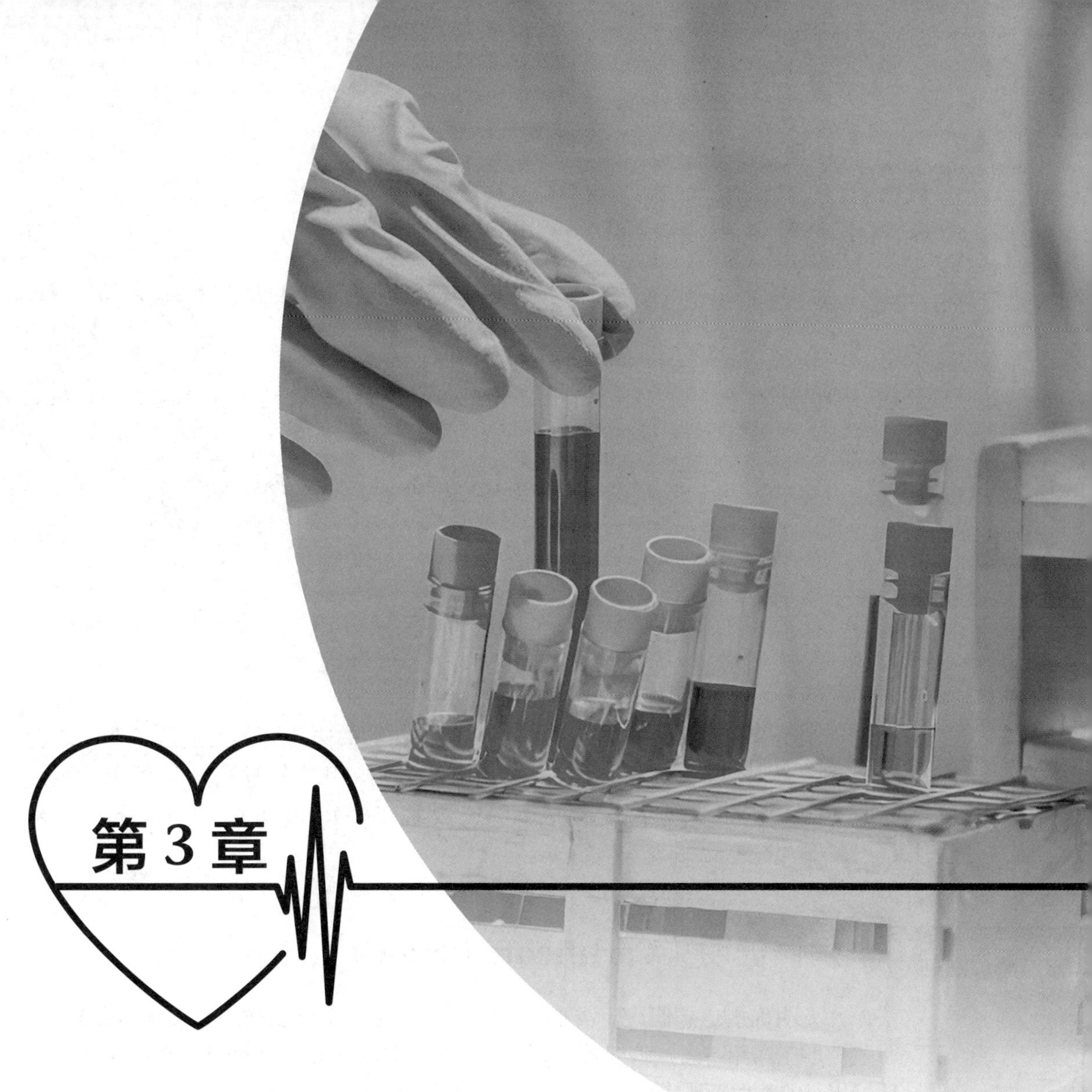

第 3 章

医 学 证 明（Medical Certificate）

Study sickness while you are well.

无病应思有病时。

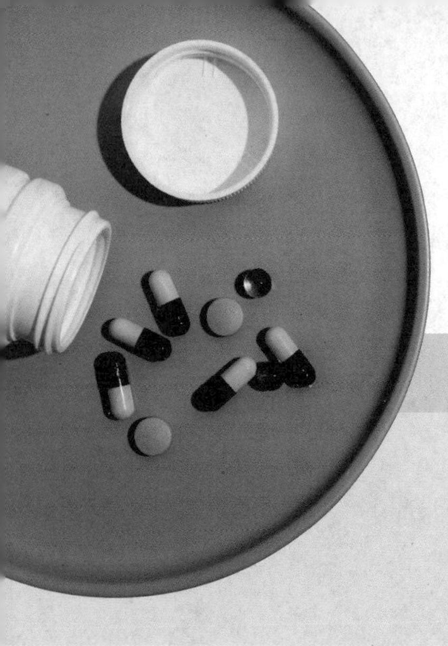

Warm-up

1. Have you heard of MC? Do you know what MC stands for?
2. In what cases are medical certificates used?

医学证明是指根据患者的需求，由具有医生执照的医生开具的病假证明，患者入院、出院、转院证明，疾病诊断证明、出生证明、死亡证明等。英语中，通常用 medical certificate 来表示医学证明，MC 经常作为 medical certificate 的缩写来使用。

3.1 病假证明（Certificate for Sick Leave）

法律并无明确规定病假一定需要医院证明。但是在实际工作中，要请带薪病假，又为了避免职工滥用带薪病假，根据用人单位的具体情况确定，通常需要提供一些证明：医院出具的病假证明书（证明书要有主治医生签名并加盖医院公章才有效）、请假条或者用人单位内部类似的其他证明。

企业职工请病假，要出具正规的医院和医疗单位开的病休证明，按照医生的建议休假时间休假，并将此证明交给单位的人事主管部门，一般要在请假当天交给单位。

【例 1】

病假证明

兹证明杨佐，女，28 岁，于 3 月 28 日被诊断为急性支气管炎。建议休息 3 天。

医生：李杰（签名）

日期：2024 年 3 月 28 日

Certificate for Sick Leave

This is to certify that Yang Zuo, female, 28 years old, was diagnosed with acute bronchitis on March 28. She is recommended to take a 3-day rest.

Doctor: Li Jie (signature)

Date: March 28, 2024

【例 2】

休假证明书

姓名：郑娜　　性别：女　　年龄：28　　科别：眼科

诊断及建议：眼睛结膜炎，眼睛发痒，烧灼，结膜充血，分泌物黏稠等；建议休息 3 天，在医生指导下使用对应的眼药水等积极进行治疗。

医师：郑有才（医院盖章）

2023 年 9 月 9 日

Leave Certificate

Name: *Zheng Na*　　Gender: *Female*　　Age: *28*

Department: *Ophthalmology*

Diagnosis and recommendations: *Conjunctivitis, itching, burning of the eyes, conjunctival congestion, thick secretions, etc. It is recommended to rest for 3 days and actively seek treatment with corresponding eye drops under the guidance of a doctor.*

Physician: *Zheng Youcai* (hospital seal)

September 9, 2023

3.2 入院证明（Admission Certificate）

住院证明一般包括入院记录、病程记录、医嘱单、辅助检查报告单和体温单等证明。现在的电子病历都会保留一段时间，去打印病历时，可以一并把出院证明打出来；如果是手写病例，可以找主治医生，说明原因后再补写一份。具有一定法律效用的医疗文件，是作为司法鉴定、保险索赔、休假等的重要依据之一。

【例 1】

入院证明

兹证明鹿鸣先生，男，73 岁，因患糖尿病，应住院进一步观察和治疗，入院时间 2023 年 5 月 9 日，住院号 3997。

主治医生：赫伯特（医院盖章）

2023 年 5 月 9 日

Admission Certificate

This is to certify that Mr. Lu Ming, male, 73 years old, suffering from diabetes, should be hospitalized for further observation and treatment. The date of admission is May 9, 2023, and the hospital number is 3997.

Surgeon-in-charge: Herbert (hospital seal)

May 9, 2023

【例 2】

XXX 省第二人民医院

入院证

门诊号：264892

姓名：毛顺　　性别：男　　年龄：62

工作单位：来顺建筑服务公司　　职业：司机

详细地址：甘肃省兰州市兰州新区秦川镇华家井村四社

入院诊断：脑梗死

入何科：内科　　☑平诊　　□急诊

费别：医保（省保、市保、新农合等）☑　　非医保□

入院日期：2023 年 10 月 6 日

医师签名：屈挺（医院专用章）

XXX Provincial Second People's Hospital

Admission Certificate

Outpatient No.: *264892*

Name: *Mao Shun*　Gender: *Male*　Age: *62*

Work unit: *Laishun Construction Service Company*

Occupation: *Driver*

Detailed address: *Group 4, Huajiajing Village, Qinchuan Town, Lanzhou New Area, Lanzhou City, Gansu Province*

Admission diagnosis: *Cerebral infarction*

Department: *Internal*　　☑ Regular Diagnosis

□ Emergency Treatment

Fee category: Medical insurance (provincial insurance, municipal insurance, new rural cooperative medical insurance, etc.) ☑　　Non-medical insurance □

Admission date: *October 6, 2023*

Physician's signature: *Qu Ting* (special seal for hospital)

3.3 转院证明（Transfer Certificate）

转院原则上是为了去更好的医院接受更好的治疗。首先，患者要到需要办理转院的医院，找到主治医生，说明情况后开具转院证明，然后拿到医院的相关部门，进行盖章；办理好之后，及时送到转院后的医院，一般情况下，医院接受转院证明的时间是有限的，所以办好证明后最好立即上交。需注意的是可能在转院途中死亡的患者不应转院。

【例】

转院证明

转诊时间：2024 年 3 月 6 日

转出医院：XXX 人民医院

转入医院：XXX 医院

患者姓名：雷兵　　性别：男　　年龄：38 岁

住址：山东省济南市 XXX 区莱蒙湖 88–1

初步诊断：肺癌

简要病史：间断咳痰、痰中带血 2 年，咯血 1 天急诊就诊。

医生签名：孙武

XXX 人民医院（盖章）

2024 年 3 月 6 日

Transfer Certificate

Referral date: *March 6, 2024*

Transferred out hospital: *XXX People's Hospital*

Transferred to hospital: *XXX Hospital*

Patient name: *Lei Bing*　　Gender: *Male*　　Age: *38*

Address: *88–1, Laimeng Lake, XXX District, Jinan, Shandong Province*

Preliminary diagnosis: *Lung cancer*

Brief medical history: *Intermittent expectoration with blood in sputum for 2 years, and 1 day of hemoptysis for emergency treatment.*

Doctor's signature: *Sun Wu*

XXX People's Hospital (hospital seal)

March 6, 2024

3.4 出院证明（Discharge Certificate）

住院患者出院时需开具出院证明，不同的医院流程可有少许差异：有些医院出院后携带住院发票、住院费用清单找主管医生即可开取；有些医院出院后携带病历、清单、诊断书找主管医生开具出院证明，去收费处盖医院公章即可。

【例】

XXX 中心医院

出院证明

山东　济南

兹证明患者穆勒先生，男，48 岁，因患疟疾，于 2023 年 12 月 9 日住院。经八天治疗后，现已痊愈，将于 2023 年 12 月 17 日出院。建议在家休息一个星期后再上班工作。

主治医生：李力（签名）

2023 年 12 月 16 日

XXX Central Hospital

Discharge Certificate

Jinan　　Shandong

This is to certify that our patient, Mr. Muller, male, aged 48, was admitted into our hospital on December 9, 2023, for malaria. After eight days of treatment, he has completely recovered and will be discharged on December 17, 2023. It is suggested that he rest for one week at home before resuming his work.

Doctor-in-charge: Li Li (signature)

December 16, 2023

3.5 疾病诊断证明（Certificate for Disease Diagnosis）

疾病诊断证明书是临床医生出具给病人用以证明其所患疾病的具有法律效用的证明文书，常常作为病休、病退、伤残鉴定、保险索赔等的重要依据。诊断证明一般包括诊断和治疗，再签上医生的名字，盖上医院的章。

【例】

山东 XXX 医院

疾病诊断证明书

编号：245892

姓名：莫宸　　性别：男　　年龄：46

科室：传染病科

住院者编号：354256

住址：济南市历下区燕子山路 15 号中国盒子小区

诊断：

1. 新型冠状病毒感染（无症状）；

2. 肺诊断性影像检查的异常所见（右肺下叶微结节）。

建议：

患者因新冠病毒感染，在我院感染科治疗。特此证明。

医生：王琳

日期：2023 年 8 月 26 日

Shandong XXX Hospital

Certificate for Disease Diagnosis

No.: 245892

Name: *Mo Chen*　　Gender: *Male*　　Age: *46*

Department: *Department of Infectious Disease*

Inpatient No.: *354256*

Address: *China Box Community, No. 15 Yanzishan Road, Lixia District, Jinan City*

Diagnosis:

1. Novel coronavirus infection (asymptomatic);

2. Abnormal findings of lung diagnostic imaging (right lower lobe nodules).

Suggestion:

The patient should receive treatment in the Department of Infectious Disease of our hospital due to COVID-19 infection. It is hereby certified.

Doctor: Wang Lin (signature)

Date: August 26, 2023

3.6 出生证明（Birth Certificate）

出生证，又被称为《出生医学证明》，是依据《中华人民共和国母婴保健法》出具的，证明婴儿出生状态、血亲关系及申报国籍、户籍从而取得公民身份的法定医学证明。出生证是每个婴儿（公民）出生都应该颁发的证件，证明其出生时间、地点、姓名、性别、体重、身高、血型、婴儿号、胎次、出生证号、健康状况、接生医生等情况。出生证是婴儿申报户口的有效证件之一。

【例】

出生公证

（2023）沪徐证外字第 123 号

兹证明吴芳，女，于一九九六年六月二十日在上海出生。吴芳的父亲是吴长斌，吴芳的母亲是李婧。

中华人民共和国上海市徐汇区公证处

公证员：何峰

二〇二三年四月一日

Notarial Certificate

(2023) L.X.Z.W.Z.NO.123

This is to certify that Wu Fang, female, was born on June 20,1996 in ShangHai. Her father is Wu Changbin and her mother is Li Jing.

Shanghai Xuhui District Notary Public Office

the People's Republic of China

Notary Public: He Feng

Dated: April 1, 2023

3.7 死亡证明（Death Certificate）

死亡证明是由合格的医生出具的法律文件，提供死者的相关身份信息，如年龄和性别，并证明死亡的时间、地点和原因。英语缩略词 DC 经常作为 Death Certificate 的缩写来使用。

【例】

死者姓名	米婷		
性别	女	民族	汉
身份证号	370211194008267954		
死亡时间	2024.4.5　21:35	年龄	84
住址	山东省青岛市黄岛经济开发区		
死亡原因	非霍奇金淋巴瘤		

（续表）

家庭成员签名			
联系方式	15678985624		
医生（签字）		户籍警察（签字）	
医院印章		当地派出所印章	

Name of the Decedent	Mi Ting		
Gender	Female	Ethnic Group	Han
ID No.	370211194008267954		
Death Time	21:35　2024.4.5	Chronological Age	84
Domicile Address	Huangdao Economic Development Zone, Qingdao City, Shandong Province		
Main Cause of Death	Non-Hodgkin lymphoma		
Signature of the Family Member			
Contact Information	15678985624		
Signature of the Doctor		Signature of the Household Registration Police	
Seal of the Medical Institute		Seal of the Local Police Station	

Exercises

Exercise I　Translate the following into English.

1. 我的健康证明丢了。
2. 医生会在病假证明上写上“接受健康监察”字样。
3. 患者应当提供医生的诊断证明。
4. 真奇怪，死亡证明上写他死于心脏衰竭。
5. 据江苏《现代快报》报道，世界杯鏖战正酣，“世界杯病假条”成为“热销商品”。

Exercise II　Translate the following into Chinese.

1. People have made a long search for the causes of malaria.
2. This is to certify that Lucy suffering from appendicitis should be admitted into our hospital for immediate operation and treatment.
3. The patient should receive treatment in the Department of Infectious Disease of our hospital due to COVID-19 infection.

Exercise III　Translate the following certificate for sick leave into English.

兹证明患者詹姆斯先生，男，36 岁，因患急性胃炎，于 2023 年 11 月 12 日住院。经 10 天治疗后，现已痊愈，将于 2023 年 11 月 22 日出院。建议在家休息一个星期后再去上班。

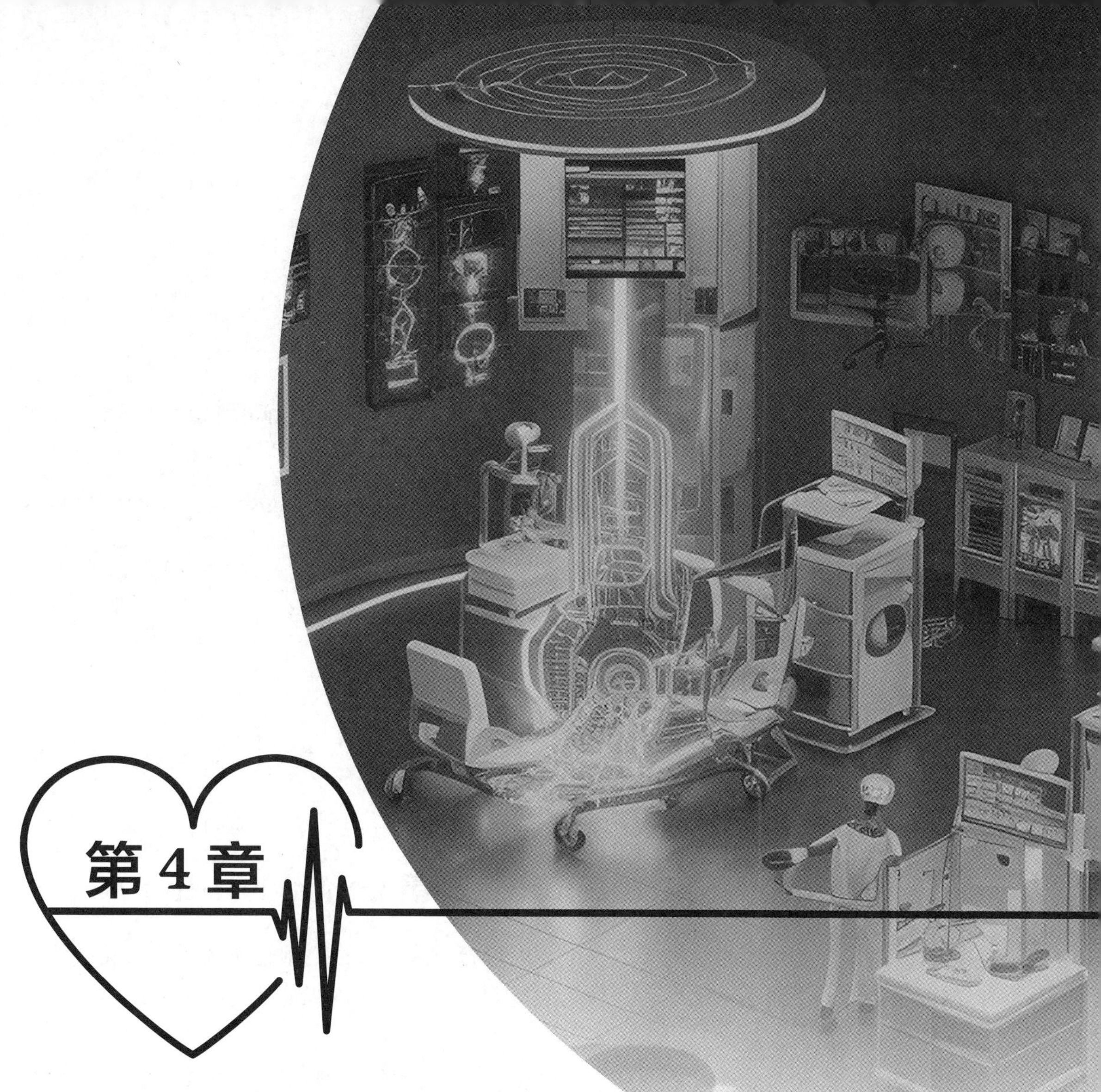

第4章

医用广告

（Medical Advertising）

Eat carrots in winter and ginger in summer, without seeking a doctor's prescription.

冬吃萝卜夏吃姜，不找医生开药方。

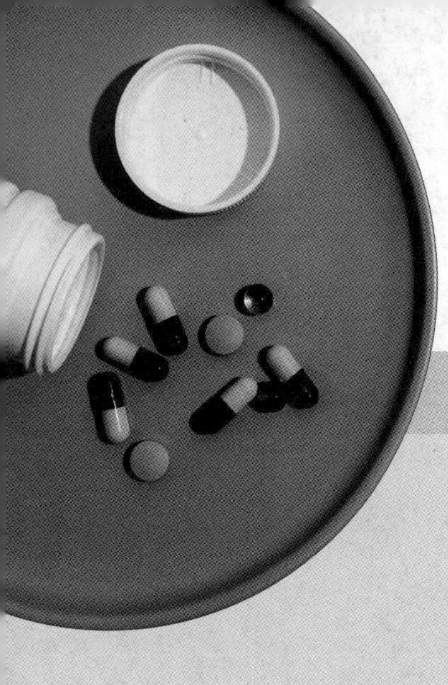

Warm-up

1. What is the medical advertising slogan that you remember the most?
2. Will you purchase medical services based on their medical advertisements?

4.1 医用广告的语言特点和分类（Language Features and Classifications of Medical Advertising）

医用广告是指医用机构等广告主体以付费方式，有计划地运用媒体将有关特殊产品或服务的信息传递给消费者，唤起消费者的注意，并说服消费者购买使用的一种信息传播活动。

医用广告关系到人民群众的身心健康和生命安全，虚假医药广告有着极大的社会危害。医用广告作为特殊服务类型的广告，受到法律法规的严格管制，发布医用广告应当符合以下要求：第一，医用广告内容必须真实、健康、科学、准确，不得以任何形式欺骗和误导公众。第二，医疗机构具有执业资格，未取得执业资格的，不得发布医用广告。第三，医用广告内容仅限于医疗机构名称、诊疗地址、从业医生姓名、技术支撑服务、商标、诊疗时间、诊疗科目、诊疗方法、通信方式。

医用广告包括医疗服务广告、医药广告、医疗器械广告、美容和药品广告等。

4.2 医疗服务广告（Medical Service Advertising）

医疗服务广告是指医疗机构，即从事疾病诊断、治疗活动的医院、卫生院、疗养院、门诊部、诊所、卫生所（室）及急救站等通过一定的媒介或者形式，向社会或者公众宣传其运用科学技术诊疗疾病的活动。

【例 1】

香港卫生署公益广告

除了专业团队、私人设备和清洁环境外，我们还需要根据《私人医疗设施条例》获得相关许可证，遵守发布的《行为准则》，并建立投诉处理机制，以保护患者的安全和权利。第一批许可证已生效。日间手术中心许可证的申请仍然开放。临床许可证和豁免书的详细信息将在稍后公布。请访问 orphf.gov.hk。

Public Service Announcement of Hong Kong Department of Health

Besides professional teams, private equipment, and clean environment, we also need to get relevant licenses under the Private Healthcare Facilities Ordinance, comply with the issue Codes of Practice, and set up a complaint handling mechanism to protect patients, safety and rights. The first batch licenses are in effect. Applications for Day Procedures Center licenses are still open. Details for clinical licenses and letters of exemption will be announced later. Please visit orphf.gov.hk.

【例 2】

拜　尔

科技创造美好生活

拜尔科学有很多方面，但有一点总是一样的，那就是改善人们的生活。我们每年在研发上花费约 30 亿欧元，雇用了 13 000 名研究人员。他们正在研究人类、动物和植物健康的解决方案。拜尔是唯一一家将这三个领域合并在一起的公司。

动物健康也是我们非常重视的问题，拜尔研发人员正致力于研发有效防治家畜、宠物病虫害的产品。我们的新产品仅需使用几滴即可对人类和动物起到数周的保护作用，令其免受虱子、跳蚤、蜱虫及疾病的侵袭。

我们一直致力于促进人类健康，心血管疾病是当今工业国家中导致死亡的最常见疾病。其中，心房颤动会导致中风，而抗凝药则能降低心房颤动患者的中风风险。癌症的治愈仍然任重而道远，我们估计全世界每天有 2 万名患者因癌症而过世。我们已经研发出一系列的新药，其中包括抑制肿瘤血液供应的活性物质。我们的研究应将继续，生物技术能够为该疾病提供新的治疗选择，我们仍将全力以赴，解决这些问题。

作为世界一流的创新型企业，我们为创造更美好的世界而不懈努力，这已经成为每天激励我们的动力。拜尔，创造美好生活。

Bayer

Science for a Better Life

Science in Bayer has many faces but one thing is always the same, improving people's lives. Every year we spend around three billion euros on research and development and we employ thirteen thousand researchers. They are working on solutions for human, animal, and plant health. Bayer is the only company to combine the three areas under one roof.

Animal health is also an issue that we attach great importance to, and Bayer R&D personnel are committed to developing products that effectively prevent and control diseases and pests in livestock and pets. Our new product can provide weeks of protection for humans and animals from lice, fleas, ticks, and diseases with just a few drops of use.

We have always been committed to promoting human health, and cardiovascular disease is the most common cause of death in industrial countries today. Atrial fibrillation can lead to strokes, while anticoagulants can reduce the risk of strokes in patients with atrial fibrillation. The cure of cancer still has a long way to go, and we estimate that 20,000 patients worldwide die from cancer every day. We have developed a series of new drugs, including active substances that inhibit tumor blood supply. Our research should continue. Biotechnology can provide new treatment options for this disease, and we will continue to do our best to address these issues.

As a world-class innovative enterprise, we strive tirelessly to create a better world, which has become our daily motivation. Bayer, create a better life.

4.3 药品广告（Pharmaceutical Advertising）

药品广告是指药品生产经营企业和医疗机构承担费用，通过一定的媒介和形式，直接或间接地介绍具体药品品种，进行以药品销售为目的的商业广告。药品广告的功能有提供药品信息，促进药品销售，树立企业品牌形象。

【例 1】

达力士

再次爱上你的皮肤

达力士牛皮癣软膏最早可在两周内缓解牛皮癣。现在可以直接从药剂师那里买到。所以，在出现突发症状的第一个迹象时，试试达力士牛皮癣软膏。确保你在镜子里看到的不是你的牛皮癣，而是你自己。

Dovonex

Love Your Skin Again

Dovonex Psoriasis Ointment provides proven relief from psoriasis in as early as two weeks. And it's now available directly from the pharmacist. So at the first sign of a flare-up, try Dovonex Psoriasis Ointment. And make sure it's not your psoriasis you see in the mirror—it's yourself.

【例 2】

维克斯昼夜感冒药

快速、强效地缓解多症状。白天使用不嗜睡的 DayQuil 缓解，晚上尝试 NyQuil 快速缓解，这样你就可以休息了。

有效缓解感冒和流感症状。DayQuil 和 NyQuil 感冒和流感药物暂时缓解普通感冒和流感症状

感觉好多了。只需一剂即可快速起效，有效缓解感冒和流感。

度过你最严重的感冒和流感症状。感冒时，生活不会停止。DayQuil 和 NyQuil 可以缓解令人烦恼的症状，如咳嗽和发烧，无论白天，还是晚上。

值得信赖的咳嗽、感冒和流感缓解：来自世界上第一个销售的非处方咳嗽和感冒品牌。125 年来，Vicks 一直被人们信任，可以缓解你最严重的感冒和流感症状。Vicks DayQuil 和 NyQuil 是第一家药剂师推荐的日间和夜间咳嗽、感冒和流感品牌。

Vicks DayQuil and NyQuil Cold & Flu LiquiCaps

Fast, powerful multi-symptom relief. Use non-drowsy DayQuil for daytime relief and at night try NyQuil for fast relief, so you can rest.

Effective cold & flu symptom relief. DayQuil and NyQuil Cold & Flu medicine temporarily relieve common cold & flu symptoms.

Feel better fast. Just one dose starts working fast to provide effective cold & flu relief.

Power through your worst cold & flu symptoms. Life doesn't stop when you have a cold. DayQuil and NyQuil relieve bothersome symptoms, such as cough and fever, day and night.

Trusted cough, cold & flu relief: From the world's first selling OTC cough and cold brand, Vicks has been trusted for over 125 years to relieve your worst cold & flu symptoms. Vicks DayQuil and NyQuil are the first pharmacist recommended daytime and nighttime cough, cold & flu brands.

4.4 医疗器械广告（Medical Device Advertising）

医疗器械广告指利用媒介或其他形式发布有关用于人体疾病诊断、治疗、预防，调节人体生理功能或替代人体器官的仪器、装置、器具、植入物、材料及相关物品的广告。

【例】

北京医疗器械检测研究所

科学检测守护健康

公正的测试 / 科学的分析 / 准确的结论 / 优质的服务

健康就是希望，健康就是责任，健康就是期望，健康也是一种无声的守护。

基于 168 个小时的环境测试和 100 多项安全和性能测试，我们相信这款超声波设备将展示生命中最感人的瞬间。

在分别进行了 500 万次疲劳和磨损测试的基础上，我们相信它可以缓解你的痛苦，让你的青春再次明亮多彩。通过其数百个参数进行测试和验证，包括电气和电磁安全元件。我们相信，该设备准确记录的生命体征是您从重病中康复的保证。

每年，我们都会对数千种产品进行测试，以确保全球医疗设备的安全使用，并保护公众健康。我们采用先进的技术进行每一次测试。我们履行对公众做出的每一项承诺。

我们将最大的热情投入我们提供的每一项服务中，并确保为每一位客户提供适当的产品质量控制。我们不断超越自我，努力提供更多、更好的服务。

我们相信，我们越努力，就越能保证医疗设备的安全使用。我们相信，我们付出的努力越大，就能创造更多的人生奇迹。

Beijing Institute of Medical Device Testing

Scientific Testing Guards Health

Fair Testing / Scientific Analysis / Accurate Conclusion / Excellent Service

Health is hope. Health is responsibility. Health is expectation. And health is also a kind of silent guardian.

Based on 168 hours of the environmental test and over 100 safety & performance tests, we believe that this ultrasound equipment will illustrate the most touching moment of life.

On the basis of 5 million cycles of fatigue and wear tests respectively, we believe that it can relieve your pain and make your youth bright and colorful again. It was tested and verified with its hundreds of parameters, including electrical and electromagnetic safety elements. We believe that the vital signs accurately recorded by this equipment are the guarantee for your recovery from serious illness.

Each year, we conduct tests to thousands of products to ensure the safe use of medical devices worldwide and to protect public health. We adopt advanced technologies to every test. We conduct and fulfill every commitment we make to the public.

We devote our greatest passion to every service we provide and to ensure proper product quality control for every client. We constantly surpass ourselves and endeavor to provide more and better services.

We believe that the greater effort we make, the more we can guarantee the safe use of medical devices. And we believe that the greater effort we make, the more miracles of life we are able to create.

4.5 美容广告（Beauty Advertising）

医疗美容是指运用手术、药物、医疗器械及其他具有创伤性或者侵入性的医学技术方法对人的容貌和人体各部位形态进行修复与再塑。使用的美容方法具有“创伤性”或者“侵入性”，是界定医疗美容的关键。医疗美容广告是指通过一定媒介或形式直接或间接介绍医疗美容机构或服务的商业广告。

【例】

（1）XXX 美容院，带给您女王级的至尊享受。

XXX Beauty Salon brings you queen level supreme enjoyment.

（2）美丽天堂：让你拥有天使脸蛋、魔鬼身材、迷人笑脸、超凡气质!

Beautiful Paradise: Let you have an angel's face, the graceful body, charming smile, and extraordinary temperament!

（3）时光从容，人生美好!

Easy in the hours, beautiful in life!

（4）世界不是缺少美丽，而是缺少修饰!

The world is not lack of beauty, but a lack of modification!

（5）无论你是谁，无论你来自哪里，无论你在这里或那里，超越所有的边界和文化；在任何年龄，在你生命中的任何时刻，在欧莱雅，我们相信美丽的力量对我们每个人来说都是如此。

Whoever you are, wherever you from, here or there, beyond all frontiers and cultures; at any age, at any moment in your life, at L'ORÉAL, we believe in the power of beauty for anyone of us.

（6）雅诗兰黛品牌宣传标语：为每个女性带来美丽。

Estée Lauder brand slogan: Bring beauty to every woman.

（7）黄金显得冰冷，钻石缺乏了生机，豪华轿车也不够吸引，不要造作，感受真实的奢华，唯有，迪奥真我香水。

Gold is cold. Diamonds are dead. A limousine is a car. Don't pretend. Feel what's real. C'est Ca Que J'adore.

（8）无论你在世界何处，我都能依香寻你。

No matter where you are in the world, I can always find you by fragrance.

Exercises

Exercise I　Translate the following into English.

1. 医用广告关系到人民群众的身心健康和生命安全，虚假医药广告有着极大的社会危害。

2. 在“互联网 +”时代，通过网络销售医药产品服务已十分普遍。

3. 国际精英、精湛技术、一流设备，为生命保驾护航。

4. 飘柔，就是这么自信。

5. 她具有无限的吸引力，闪烁着耀眼的光辉，真正的优雅品位。（古龙香水）

Exercise II　Translate the following into Chinese.

1. Today's Mindray medical products are exported to over 190 countries and regions worldwide and widely used in top hospitals worldwide.

2. For global medical device companies, they are faced with similar problems, namely rapid product technology updates and iteration + ceiling effects in segmented fields.

3. The ability to master cutting-edge technologies in segmented fields often becomes the key to whether a company can sustain its market share.

Exercise III　Translate the following medical device advertising into English.

山东道尔格医疗器械制造有限公司，是一家专注于高端专业医疗器械经营销售的大型现代化企业。多年来，公司一直坚持以客户需求为核心、以精品为导向，为客户提供医疗器械的整体解决方案；坚持“领先科技，传递梦想”的理念，为客户提供高科技产品，帮助医生更快、更安全地为大众服务，传递健康梦想。

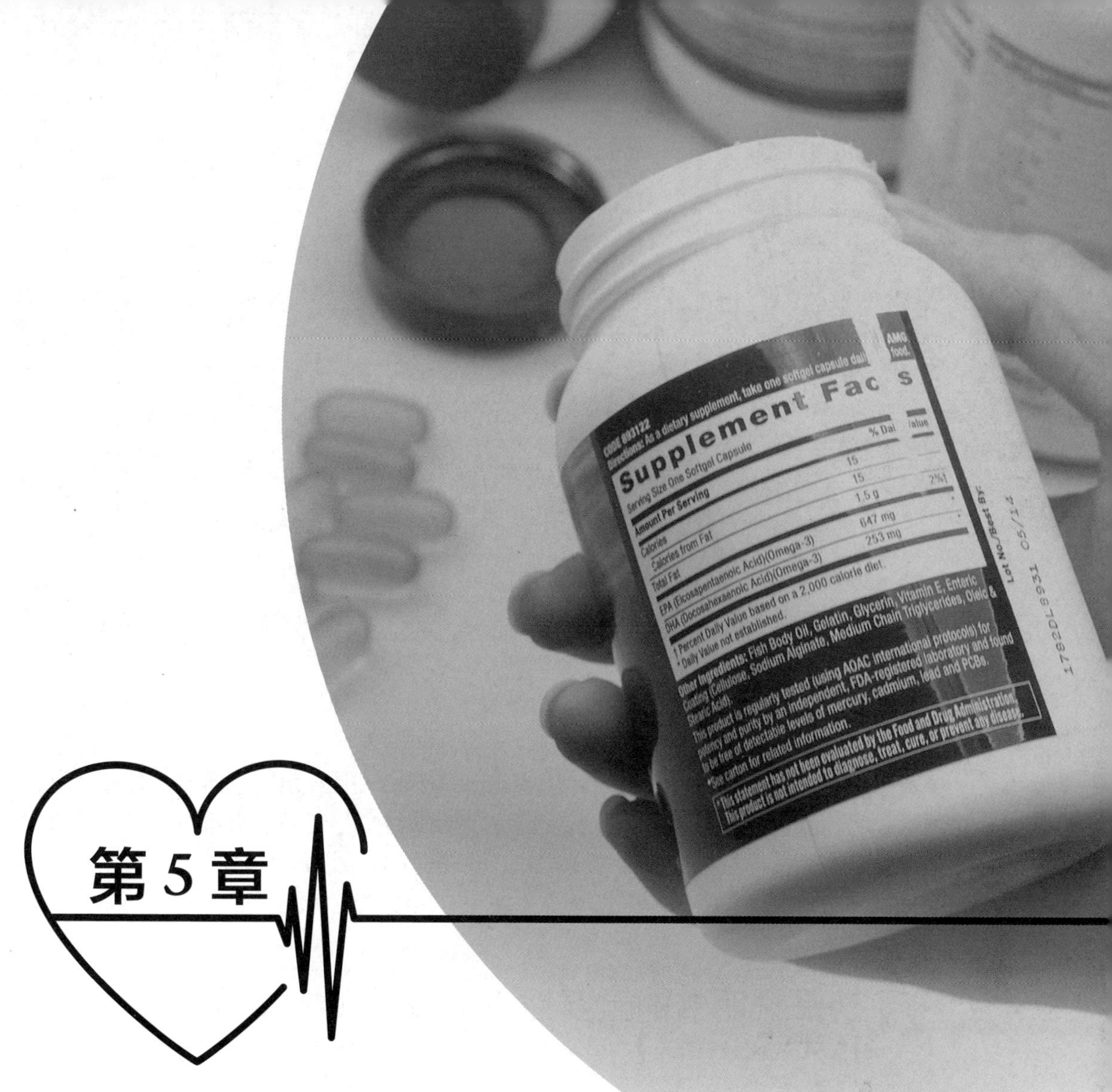

第5章

药品说明书
（Drug Instructions）

Bitter pills may have wholesome effects.

良药苦口利于病。

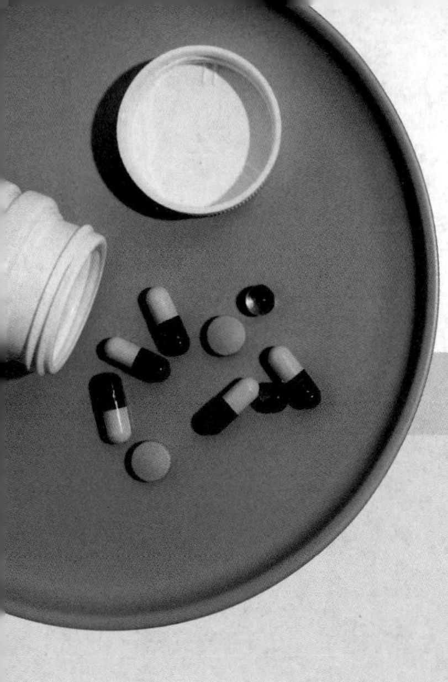

Warm-up

1. What do you want to know before you take medicine?
2. What is your experience of medicine prescriptions?
3. What are the risks of self-medication?

药品说明书（Drug Instructions / Package Insert）是经由国家药品监督管理部门核准、载明药品重要信息的管理文件。药品说明书包含与药品使用相关的和必要的医学信息，是药品情况说明的重要来源之一，也是医师、药师、护师和患者治疗及用药时的重要依据。

5.1 药品说明书的重要性（Importance of Drug Instructions）

药品说明书的受众广泛，不但有医师、药师、护师等专业医护人员，更包括药品实际使用者——患者及患者家属等欠缺医药学专业背景的人士。因此，药品说明书既要体现其专业性，又要做到易于阅读，使人准确理解药品的用法、用量及相关的注意事项。

5.2 药品说明书的基本构成（Basic Composition of Drug Instructions）

根据我国 2022 年发布的《化学药品及生物制品说明书通用格式和撰写指南》，药品说明书的内容应包括：警示语、药品名称、适应症、规格、用法用量、不良反应、禁忌、注意事项、贮藏、包装、有效期、执行标准、批准文号、生产企业等项目。作为重要的药品说明文件，药品说明书经由国家药品质量监管部门核准上市，是药品包装中必不可少的一部分。虽然《中华人民共和国药品管理法》对药品说明书做出了详细规定，但在具体使用中，大多数刚刚进入医疗行业的从业人员及广大患者，对于药品说明书的理解依旧是较为困难的事情。本章结合我国化学药品非处方药说明书规范细则，并参考美国食品药品监督管理局（FDA）的相关法规，对药品说明书分部分进行阐述。

5.2.1 警示语（Warnings）

《化学药品及生物制品说明书通用格式和撰写指南》对“警示语”定义如下：“警示语”是指药品严重不良反应（可导致死亡或严重伤害）及其严重安全性问题警告的摘要，可涉及禁忌和注意事项等项目的内容。这些内容应当在说明书标题下以醒目的黑体字注明。若无相关内容，不列该项。目前，我国的药品说明书中，对于警示语部分虽有一些原则性的规定，但并不是所有的药品说明书都包含警示语部分。在本章节，我们部分参考了美国食品药品监督管理局的相关法规，对警示语部分加以说明。

【例 1】

Benzylpenicillin Sodium for Injection

Please read the insert carefully before use, or buy and use the product under pharmacist's instructions.

Prohibited for patients with penicillin allergy history or positive skin test reaction.

注射用青霉素钠说明书

请仔细阅读说明书并按说明使用或在医师指导下购买和使用。

有青霉素类药物过敏史或青霉素皮肤试验阳性患者禁用。

以类风湿性关节炎常用药美洛昔康（Meloxicam）为例，美国食品药品监督管理局批准的美洛昔康片剂说明书中明确告知了使用者有关严重心血管及胃肠事件风险。该药品警示语如下：

【例 2】

WARNING: RISK OF SERIOUS CARDIOVASCULAR AND GASTROINTESTINAL EVENTS

See full prescribing information for complete boxed warning.

Nonsteroidal anti-inflammatory drugs (NSAIDs) cause an increased risk of serious cardiovascular thrombotic events, including myocardial infarction and strokes, which can be fatal. This risk may occur early in treatment and may increase with duration of use (5.1).

Meloxicam is contraindicated in the setting of coronary artery bypass graft (CABG) surgery (4, 5.1).

NSAIDs cause an increased risk of serious gastrointestinal (GI) adverse events including bleeding, ulceration, and perforation of the stomach or intestines, which can be fatal. These events can occur at any time during use and without warning symptoms. Elderly patients and patients with a prior history of peptic ulcer disease and/or GI bleeding are at greater risk for serious GI events (5.2).

警告：严重心血管和胃肠道事件的风险

有关完整的黑框警告，请参阅完整的处方信息。

非甾体类抗炎药（NSAIDs）会增加严重心血管血栓事件的风险，包括心肌梗死和中风，此类症状可能是致命的。这种风险可能在治疗早期发生，并可能随着该药物使用时间的延长而增加（5.1）。

美洛昔康禁用于冠状动脉搭桥（CABG）术（4，5.1）。

非甾体抗炎药会增加严重胃肠道（GI）不良事件的风险，包括出血、溃疡和胃肠穿孔，此类症状可能是致命的。这些情况可能在药物使用过程中的任何时间发生，并且不会出现患病先兆。老年患者和有消化性溃疡病史和/或胃肠道出血史的患者发生严重胃肠道症状的风险更大（5.2）。

美国食品药品监督管理局药品说明书中有两处警示语：一处是在说明书开始、以黑框的形式框出的警告语；另一处则体现在药品完整的处方信息中。

警示语是药品说明书中不可忽视的一部分，忽视警示语有可能导致患者的健康受损，甚至危及其生命。作为医务工作者，更应对药品说明书中警示语的部分多加注意。

5.2.2 药品名称（Drug Names）

在药品说明书中，药品名称可分为通用名称（Approved Drug Name / Generic Name）、商品名称（Trade Name / Proprietary Name）、英文名称及汉语拼音。在我国，药品的通用名称（China Approved Drug Names）是由国家药典委员会（Chinese Pharmacopoeia Commission）依照国家相关法规组织制定，并报国家药品监督管理局备案的药品的法定名称，也是在该药品外包装和说明书上必须标注的名称；国内药品说明书通常会在通用名称后标注药品的商品名称、英文名称及汉语拼音。药品的通用名称在一定程度上反映了该药品的主要有效成份，但绝不可用于商标注册。药品的商品名称是药品生产厂家为销售药品而注册的、便于消费者识记的名称。同一种药品由不同的药品生产厂家生产，其化学名称和通用名称可以相同，但商品名称必然不同。

例如，由多家制药公司生产的同一类药品，它们的通用名称均可标注为阿莫西林胶囊（Amoxicillin Capsules），制药公司也可为其注册不同的商品名称，以便销售本公司生产的药品。药品商品名称的右上角（或左上角）标注有 ® 的标记。® 是 Register（注册）的缩写，药品说明书中有此标识，表示该药品已通过国家药品监督管理部门核准，取得了专用的注册商标（Registered Trade Mark）。

5.2.3 成份（Ingredients）与性状（Description）

在药品说明书中，“成份”一栏一般由以下部分组成：化学名称（Chemical Name）、化学结构式（Structural Formula）、分子式（Molecular Formula）和分子量（Molecular Weight）。药品说明书中的药物化学名称可以体现该药品的化学结构组成成份。若药品的化学名称很长，我们可以把化学名称分解开，查询各部分的名称之后再进行组合。根据药物的不同种类，有些说明书中只标注药品生产所用的主料和辅料，如中成药。药品的“性状”一栏则体现了该药的外观、颜色、气味等物理特征或形态。

1. 常用表达

1）词汇

gas 气体	liquid 液体	solid 固体	power 粉末
solution 溶液	soluble 可溶的	insoluble 不溶的	solubility 溶解度
tasteless 无味的	colorless 无色的	odorless 无臭的	odor 气味
crystalline 结晶的	sterile 无菌的	derivative 衍生物	excipient 辅料
compound 化合物		molecular formula 分子式	
molecular weight 分子量			

2）句型

be derived from 由……衍生

consist of 由……组成

contain 含有

be prepared from 由……制备

be soluble in 溶于……

3）例句

（1）Compound A is a colorless or white crystal.

化合物 A 为无色或白色结晶。

（2）Compound B is a pastel yellow crystalline powder which is odorless and hygroscopic.

化合物 B 是一种淡黄色结晶粉末且具有吸湿性。

（3）Compound C is very soluble/insoluble in water.

化合物 C 极易 / 极不易溶于水。

（4） The pH of the reconstituted product is between 5.0 and 7.5.

重组产物的 pH 值在 5.0 和 7.5 之间。

（5） The compound has the following structural formula.

该化合物具有以下结构式。

（6） Methylphenidate hydrochloride is a white, odorless, fine crystalline powder. Its solutions are acid to litmus.

盐酸哌甲酯是一种白色、无味、精细的结晶粉末，其溶液对石蕊呈酸性。

（7） Meloxicam is a pastel yellow solid, practically insoluble in water, with higher solubility observed in strong acids and bases.

美洛昔康是一种淡黄色固体，几乎不溶于水，在强酸和强碱中具有较高的溶解度。

（8） Nitroglycerin, an organic nitrate, is a vasodilator which has effects on both arteries and veins.

硝酸甘油是一种有机硝酸盐，是一种血管扩张剂，对动脉和静脉都有作用。

（9） This product delivers nitroglycerin in the form of spray droplets onto or under the tongue.

该产品以喷雾液滴的形式将硝酸甘油输送至舌上或舌下。

（10）Methylphenidate is a mild central nervous system (CNS) stimulant, available as 2.5 mg, 5 mg and 10 mg chewable tablets for oral administration.

盐酸哌甲酯是一种温和的中枢神经系统（CNS）兴奋剂，有 2.5 mg、5 mg 和 10 mg 的咀嚼片供口服。

（11）It is freely soluble in water and in methanol, soluble in alcohol, and slightly soluble in chloroform and in acetone.

它易溶于水和甲醇，溶于乙醇，微溶于氯仿和丙酮。

（12）It may be used alone or with other medications.

它可单独使用或与其他药物一起使用。

（13）It is not known if... is safe and effective in children younger than six months of age.

目前尚不清楚……对六个月以下的儿童是否安全有效。

（14）The capsules are intended for oral administration.

此类胶囊用于口服。

（15）Aqueous solutions of folic acid are heat sensitive and rapidly decompose in the presence of light. It should be stored in a cool place protected from light.

叶酸水溶液对热敏感并在光照下迅速分解，其溶液应避光保存在阴凉处。

（16）Fentanyl buccal tablets are an opioid agonist, intended for buccal mucosal administration.

芬太尼含片是一种阿片类激动剂，用于口腔黏膜给药。

2. 示例

【例 1】

Description: Buffered Pfizerpen (penicillin G potassium) for Injection is a sterile, pyrogen-free powder for reconstitution. Buffered Pfizerpen (penicillin G potassium) for Injection is an antibacterial agent for intramuscular, continuous intravenous drip, intrapleural or other local infusion.

Each million unit contains approximately 6.8 milligrams of sodium (0.3 mEq) and 65.6 milligrams of potassium (1.68 mEq).

Penicillin G potassium is a colorless or white crystal, or a white crystalline powder which is odorless, or practically so, and moderately hygroscopic. Penicillin G potassium is very soluble in water.

描述：由辉瑞提供的注射用青霉素 G 钾缓冲液是一种无菌无热原的重构粉末，是一种抗菌剂，用于肌注、连续静脉滴注、胸膜内或其他局部注射。

每百万单位约含 6.8 毫克钠（0.3 Eq）和 65.6 毫克钾（1.68 Eq）。

青霉素 G 钾为无色 / 白色晶体或无色结晶粉末，无臭或几乎无臭，且具有适度吸湿性。青霉素 G 钾极易溶于水。

【例 2】

Lianhua Qingwen Capsules

Ingredients: Weeping Forsythia, Honeysuckle Flower, Ephedra Herb (honey-fried), Bitter Apricot Seed (stir-baked), Gypsum, Isatis Root, Male Fern Rhizome, Heartleaf Houttuynia Herb, Cablin Patchouli Herb, Rhubarb, Bigflower Rhodiola Root, Menthol, Liquorice Root. Excipient: Starch.

Description: Capsules, containing tan to brown granules and powders; odor, slightly aromatic; taste, slightly bitter.

连花清瘟胶囊

成份：连翘、金银花、炙麻黄、炒苦杏仁、石膏、板蓝根、绵马贯众、鱼腥草、广藿香、大黄、红景天、薄荷脑、甘草。辅料：淀粉。

性状：胶囊，内容物为棕黄色至黄褐色的颗粒和粉末；气微香，味微苦。

5.2.4 适应症（Indication）

在药品说明书中，“适应症”一栏中体现的内容可以使医护人员明确地找到适合患者的治疗方法。《化学药品及生物制品说明书通用格式和撰写指南》中明确说明：“应当根据该药品的用途，采用准确的表述方式，明确用于预防、治疗、诊断、缓解或者辅助治疗某种疾病（状态）或者症状。”

1. 常用表达

be administered in 适用于

be effective in/for/against 对……有效

be active against 对……有效

be recommended for 推荐用于

be employed to / be used to / be helpful in / be useful in 用于

be associated/combined with 与……合用

2. 示例

以吸入用布地奈德混悬液（Budesonide Suspension for Inhalation）为例，该药品是一种治疗支气管哮喘的气雾剂，有着明确的患者群和使用年龄限制，在药品说明书中的“适应症”一栏中的体现如下：

【例】

Budesonide Suspension for Inhalation is an inhaled corticosteroid indicated for:

Maintenance treatment of asthma and as prophylactic therapy in children 12 months to 8 years of age.

布地奈德混悬液是一种吸入皮质类固醇，适用于：

哮喘的维持治疗和作为 12 个月至 8 岁儿童的预防性治疗。

该药品说明书的“适应症”一栏明确了其在哮喘中的治疗价值及适用的患者年龄段，并且指明该药适用于治疗及预防性治疗。这样的描述使得医务人员和患者家属在药品选择上更加慎重。

5.2.5 药品规格及用法用量（Drug Specification/Dosage and Administration）

在药品说明书中，药品规格及用法用量不仅是医师确定给药的重要依据，也是护士执行给药过程、患者自行服药的重要凭据。《中华人民共和国药典（二部 2020 年版）》

凡例第 20 条将化学药制剂规格解释为：系指每一支、片或其他每一个单位制剂中含有主药的重量（或效价）或含量（%）或装量。用法用量是指药品的使用方法及在一定时间内服用该药品的数量。《化学药品及生物制品说明书通用格式和撰写指南》中规定："【用法用量】应包括用法和用量两部分。需按疗程用药或者规定用药期限的，必须注明疗程、期限。应当详细列出该药品的用药方法，准确列出用药频次、用药剂量以及疗程期限，并应当特别注意剂量与规格的关系。用法上有特殊要求的，应当按实际情况详细说明。"

1. 常用表达

1）词汇

- **dosage form 剂型**

tablet 片剂 | capsule 胶囊剂 | pill 丸剂
granule 冲剂 / 颗粒剂 | powder 粉剂 | injection 注射剂
ointment 软膏剂 | cream 乳膏剂 | paste 糊剂
syrup 糖浆剂 | solution 溶液剂 | emulsion 乳剂
suspension 混悬剂 | suppository 栓剂 | aerosol 气雾剂
pellicle 薄膜剂 | drop 滴剂 | decoction 汤剂
paint 涂剂 | tincture 酊剂 | mucilage 胶浆剂
mixture 合剂 | honeyed bolus 蜜丸
sublingual tablet 舌下片剂 | concentrated pill 浓缩丸

- **unit of measurement 计量单位**

kilogram (kg) 千克 | gram (g) 克 | milligram (mg) 毫克
microgram (mcg) 微克 | liter (L) 升 | milliliter (mL) 毫升
unit 单位 | percent (%) 百分比
international unit (IU) 国际单位
million international unit (MIU) 百万国际单位
Klobusitzky unit (KU) 克氏单位

- **route of administration 给药途径**

per os (by mouth) 口服
by sublingually 含服 / 舌下给药
by intravenous injection (IV) 静脉注射
by subcutaneous injection (SC) 皮下注射
by intradermal injection (ID) 皮内注射

by intramuscular injection (IM) 肌肉注射

by intragastric administration (IG) 灌胃

by enema/clyster 灌肠

by aerosol 气雾剂

by inhalation (INH) 雾化吸入

- **administration method 给药方法**

take 服用
swallow 吞服
inject 注射
inhale 吸入
spray 喷雾
apply to 涂抹

- **dosage 剂量**

overdose 过量
average dose 平均剂量
divided dose 分次剂量
minimum dose 最小剂量
maximum dose 最大剂量
fatal dose 致死剂量
single dose 单次剂量
multiple dose 多次剂量
daily dose 单日剂量
initial/beginning/starting dose 首次剂量
indicated dose 有效剂量
standard dose 标准剂量
suggested/recommended dose 推荐剂量
normal dose 常用剂量

- **times of administer drug 给药次数**

per day / a day / every day 每日

every... hours 每隔……小时

once/twice a day / daily 每日一 / 两次

three times a day /daily 每日三次

every other day 每隔一日

intervals of 每隔……

once/twice a week / weekly 每周一 / 两次

three times a week 每周三次

divided into... doses 分……次

in two/three divided doses 分两次 / 三次剂量

- **target of administration 给药对象**

adult 成年人
male 男性
female 女性
adolescent 青少年
infant 婴幼儿
elderly patient 老年患者
newborn baby 新生儿
pregnant woman 孕妇

2）缩写

处方中的常用拉丁语缩写如表 5.1 所示：

表 5.1　处方中常用拉丁语缩写

Abbreviation	Chinese
p.o.	口服
p.c.	饭后
a.c.	饭前
b.i.d.	每日两次
t.i.d.	每日三次
q.i.d.	每日四次
q.o.d.	隔日一次
q.h.	每小时一次
q.a.m.	上午一次
q.n.	每晚一次
b.i.w.	每周两次
i.m.	肌肉注射
ad us.int.	内服
ad us.ext.	外用
i.v.	静脉注射
inhal.	吸入剂
Rp.	请取

3）例句

（1）It was approved to treat for adults and pediatric patients at least 12 years of age.

此药物被批准用于成人及 12 岁以上的儿科患者。

（2）The average daily dose is 1 pill 3 times daily.

每天服药剂量为一天 3 次，一次 1 片。

（3） It is advisable to initiate therapy with massive doses.

开始治疗时，建议加大用量。

（4） It is recommended that the dose be reduced.

建议减少用量。

（5） Avoid irritation of...

应避免……刺激。

（6） Treatment is administered for 3 to 7 days.

疗程持续 3 ~ 7 天。

（7） Care should be taken to ensure that... are not crushed or chewed or retained in the mouth.

应注意确保……不会被压碎、咀嚼或留在嘴里。

（8） The usual dose of oral... is 50 mg every 8 hours, but a dose of 150 mg every 24 hours may be administered.

通常情况下，口服……的剂量为每 8 小时服药 50 毫克，也可以每 24 小时服药 150 毫克。

（9） The recommended total daily dose for pediatric patients is 15 to 30 mg/kg given in equally divided doses for 3 to7 days.

对于儿科患者，推荐的每日总剂量为 15 ~ 30 毫克 / 千克 , 分等剂量给药，持续 3 ~ 7 天。

（10）In the treatment of... duration of at least 14 days is recommended.

在治疗……时，建议持续治疗至少 14 天。

（11）In severe infections, a total daily dose of 50 to 100 mg/kg may be administered in equally divided doses.

治疗严重感染时，每日用药总剂量为 50 ~ 100 毫克 / 千克，等分剂量给药。

（12）For the treatment of... the recommended daily dose is 50 to 100 mg/kg given in equally divided doses.

对于……的治疗，建议每日剂量为 50 ~ 100 毫克 / 千克，等分剂量给药。

（13）A white powder filled into an opaque white and opaque dark blue capsule that is imprinted with... 150 mg in edible black ink on the white body.

在不透明的蓝白胶囊包装中填充白色粉末，并用可食用黑墨水在胶囊白色部分注明……150 毫克字样。

（14）The capsules and oral suspension may be taken with or without food; however, tolerability may be enhanced if it is taken with food.

胶囊和口服混悬液可随餐服用，亦可不随餐服用；若随餐服用，或可增强耐受性。

（15）The capsules are to be taken before or after a meal with a little water.

胶囊应于饭前或饭后用少量水送服。

（16）The recommended dose of... in adult patients with acute uncomplicated influenza is a single 300 mg dose.

对于患有急性无并发症流感的成年人，……推荐剂量为单次 300 毫克。

（17）However, coadministration of... with dairy products or oral supplements (e.g., calcium, iron, magnesium, selenium, or zinc) should be avoided.

然而，应避免……与乳制品或口服补剂（如钙、铁、镁、硒或锌）同时服用。

（18）More severe infections were caused, particularly those due to proven streptococci, pneumococci, and staphylococci: a minimum of 5 million units daily.

造成了更严重的感染，尤其是被证实由链球菌、肺炎球菌和葡萄球菌而引起的感染，每天至少（用药）500 万单位。

（19）Doses over the recommended daily intake level of 500 mg/day have been associated with an increased risk of...

超过推荐的摄入量 500 毫克 / 天的剂量会增加患……的风险。

2. 示例

【例 1】

Yosprala (aspirin and omeprazole) delayed-release tablets, for oral use.

Recommended dosage: One tablet daily at least 60 minutes before a meal. Do not split, chew, crush, or dissolve the tablet.

Yosprala（阿司匹林和奥美拉唑）缓释片，口服。

推荐剂量：每日一粒，至少于饭前 60 分钟服用。不要掰开、咀嚼、压碎或溶解药片。

【例 2】

Levofloxacin tablets, USP 250 mg are pink colored, capsule shaped, biconvex...

Levofloxacin tablets, USP 500 mg are orange colored, capsule shaped, biconvex...

Levofloxacin tablets, USP 750 mg are white colored, capsule shaped, biconvex...

左氧氟沙星，250 毫克，粉红色，胶囊状双凸面片剂……

左氧氟沙星，500 毫克，橙色，胶囊状双凸面片剂……

左氧氟沙星，750 毫克，白色，胶囊状双凸面片剂……

该药品的用法用量参照表 5.2：

Table 5.2 Dosage in adult patients with normal renal function

Type of Infection	Dosed Every 24 Hours	Duration (Days)
Nosocomial Pneumonia	750 mg	7–14
Community Acquired Pneumonia	500 mg	7–14
	750 mg	5
Complicated Skin and Skin Structure Infections (SSSI)	750 mg	7–14
Uncomplicated SSSI	500 mg	7–10
Chronic Bacterial Prostatitis	500 mg	28
Complicated Urinary Tract Infection (CUTI) or Acute Pyelonephritis (AP)	750 mg	5
Uncomplicated Urinary Tract Infection	250 mg	3
Acute Bacterial Exacerbation of Chronic Bronchitis (ABECB)	500 mg	7
Acute Bacterial Sinusitis (ABS)	750 mg	5
	500 mg	10–14

表 5.2 肾功能正常的成年患者使用剂量

感染类型	每 24 小时给药剂量	持续给药时间（天）
院内获得性肺炎	750 毫克	7 ~ 14
社区获得性肺炎	500 毫克	7 ~ 14
	750 毫克	5
复杂性皮肤及皮肤结构感染	750 毫克	7 ~ 14
非复杂性皮肤及皮肤结构感染	500 毫克	7 ~ 10
慢性细菌性前列腺炎	500 毫克	28

（续表）

<table>
<tr><th>感染类型</th><th>每 24 小时给药剂量</th><th>持续给药时间（天）</th></tr>
<tr><td>并发性尿路感染或急性肾盂肾炎</td><td>750 毫克</td><td>5</td></tr>
<tr><td>非复杂性尿路感染</td><td>250 毫克</td><td>3</td></tr>
<tr><td>慢性支气管炎的急性细菌性发作</td><td>500 毫克</td><td>7</td></tr>
<tr><td rowspan="2">急性细菌性鼻窦炎</td><td>750 毫克</td><td>5</td></tr>
<tr><td>500 毫克</td><td>10 ~ 14</td></tr>
</table>

5.2.6 不良反应（Adverse Reactions）与副作用（Side Effects）

药物的不良反应，顾名思义，是指药品在按照正常用法和用量的使用过程中，出现了与治疗目的无关的不良事件。不良反应既包括处方药的不良反应，也包括药物在临床试验时发生的不良反应及药品消费者等主动发起的自发报告的不良反应。这三者在药品说明书"不良反应"一栏中依次体现。药物的副作用、毒性作用、过敏反应、继发性反应等均属药物的不良反应。

药物的副作用是指在按照药品治疗剂量使用后出现的、与治疗目的无关的药理作用，是药物不良反应中的一种。在服用同样剂量的同种药物时，不同患者可能出现不同的副作用。有时，药品说明书中"副作用"部分会与"警示语"部分合为一项。

1. 常用表达

1）与不良反应相关的词汇

adverse reactions / unwanted reactions / untoward reactions 不良反应

side effects / side reactions / unwanted effects / undesirable effects 副作用

allergic reactions / hypersensitive reactions / anaphylactic reactions 过敏反应

allergic/hypersensitive/anaphylactic 过敏的

toxicity 毒性　　toxic effects 毒性反应

tolerate 耐受　　tolerance 耐受性

acute 急性的　　chronic 慢性的

common 常见的　　normal 正常的

rare 罕见的　　mild 轻微的

reversible 可逆的　　irreversible 不可逆的

severe 严重的
temporary 暂时的
secondary response 继发性反应
result from 由……引起
result in 导致
be caused by 导致

2）常见副作用

- **gastrointestinal experiences 胃肠道反应**

abdominal pain 腹痛
constipation 便秘
diarrhea 腹泻
dyspepsia 消化不良
flatulence 胃肠胀气
gross bleeding 大出血
perforation 穿孔
heartburn 胃灼热
nausea 恶心
vomiting 呕吐
GI ulcer (gastric/duodenal) 胃肠道溃疡（胃 / 十二指肠）

- **cardiovascular system 心血管系统**

hypertension 高血压
hypotension 低血压
tachycardia 心动过速
arrhythmia 心律失常
syncope 晕厥
palpitations 心悸
vasculitis 血管炎
congestive heart failure 充血性心力衰竭
myocardial infarction 心肌梗死

- **digestive system 消化系统**

esophagitis 食管炎
gastritis 胃炎
glossitis 舌炎
hematemesis 呕血
hepatitis 肝炎
jaundice 黄疸
nausea 恶心
colitis 结肠炎
eructation 嗳气
pancreatitis 胰腺炎
liver failure 肝功能衰竭
liver necrosis 肝坏死
dry mouth 口干
gastric/peptic ulcer 胃 / 消化性溃疡
gastrointestinal bleeding 消化道出血

- **hemic and lymphatic system 血液和淋巴系统**

ecchymosis 瘀斑
eosinophilia 嗜酸性粒细胞增多
leucopenia 白细胞减少
melena 黑便
purpura 紫癜
stomatitis 口腔炎
agranulocytosis 粒细胞缺乏症
lymphadenopathy 淋巴结病
pancytopenia 全血细胞减少症
thrombocytopenia 血小板减少

hemolytic anemia 溶血性贫血
aplastic anemia 再生障碍性贫血
rectal bleeding 直肠出血

- **metabolism and nutrition 代谢和营养**

hyperglycemia 高血糖
weight change 体重变化

- **nervous system 神经系统**

anxiety 焦虑
asthenia 乏力
confusion 精神错乱
depression 抑郁
drowsiness/somnolence 嗜睡
insomnia 失眠
malaise 不适
nervousness 紧张
paresthesia 感觉异常
tremor 震颤
vertigo 眩晕
spasm 痉挛
convulsion 抽搐
coma 昏迷
hallucination 幻觉
meningitis 脑膜炎
dream abnormality 梦境异常

- **respiratory system 呼吸系统**

asthma 哮喘
dyspnea 呼吸困难
pneumonia 肺炎
respiratory depression 呼吸抑制

- **skin and appendage 皮肤及附件**

alopecia 脱发
photosensitivity 光过敏
sweating 出汗
flush 潮红
pruritus 瘙痒
rash 皮疹
urticaria 荨麻疹

- **special sense 特殊感官**

blurred vision 视力模糊
conjunctivitis 结膜炎
hearing impairment 听力障碍

- **urogenital system 泌尿生殖系统**

cystitis 膀胱炎
dysuria 排尿困难
hematuria 血尿
oliguria 少尿
polyuria 多尿
proteinuria 蛋白尿
renal failure 肾功能衰竭
interstitial nephritis 间质性肾炎

3）常用句型

（1） This drug is generally well tolerated.

这种药物通常具有良好的耐受性。

（2） The most frequently reported drug related adverse reaction was...

最常报告的药物相关不良反应是……

（3） The commonest side effects associated with it are...

与之相关的最常见的副作用是……

（4） Ascorbic acid may cause serious side effects including nausea, vomiting, heartburn, stomach cramps, and headaches.

抗坏血酸可能会导致严重的副作用，包括恶心、呕吐、胃灼热、胃痉挛、头痛。

（5） Side-effects are rare with...

……的副作用很罕见。

（6） Penicillin G is relatively nontoxic, and dosage adjustments are generally required only in cases of severe renal impairment.

青霉素 G 相对无毒，通常只有在严重肾功能损害的情况下才需要调整剂量。

（7） The most commonly occurring adverse events in celecoxib treated patients were headache, fever, abdominal pain, nausea, arthralgia, diarrhea, and vomiting.

使用塞来昔布治疗时，患者最常见的不良反应为头痛、发热、腹痛、恶心、关节痛、腹泻和呕吐。

（8） Transient mild soreness may occur at the site of intramuscular or subcutaneous injection.

肌肉或皮下注射部位可能会出现短暂的轻微酸痛。

（9） Too-rapid intravenous administration of the solution may cause temporary faintness or dizziness.

静脉给药注射过快可能会导致暂时性昏厥或头晕。

（10）Caution should be exercised in patients with signs and symptoms of hepatic impairment who are being treated with potentially hepatotoxic drugs.

对于有肝功能损害症状和体征的患者，在接受潜在的肝毒性药物进行治疗时应谨慎。

（11）The reaction begins one hour after initiation of therapy and disappears within seven hours.

该反应在治疗开始后一小时出现，并在七小时内消失。

（12）These unwanted effects usually disappear after 24 hours.

此类副作用通常在 24 小时后消失。

（13）Immediate reactions usually occur within 15 minutes.

立即反应通常在（给药后）15 分钟内发生。

（14）Delayed reactions to penicillin therapy usually occur within 1–2 weeks after initiation of therapy.

青霉素治疗的延迟反应通常发生在治疗开始后 1 ~ 2 周内。

（15）Some patients discontinued therapy due to these adverse reactions.

一些患者由于这些不良反应而停止治疗。

（16）Females and patients under 25 years old experienced a higher incidence of Medical K-associated visual adverse reactions.

女性及 25 岁以下的患者使用时，与 K 药品相关的视觉障碍发生率较高。

（17）Clostridium difficile associated diarrhea (CDAD) has been reported with use of nearly all antibacterial agents, and may range in severity from mild diarrhea to fatal colitis.

几乎所有抗菌药物都会导致艰难梭菌相关性腹泻，其严重程度可能从轻度腹泻到致命性结肠炎不等。

（18）Serious adverse reactions have been reported in patients taking A concomitantly with B.

在同时服用 A 药 和 B 药的患者中报告了严重的不良反应。

（19）... is contraindicated in patients with a personal or family history of MTC (Medullary Thyroid Carcinoma).

……禁用于有甲状腺髓样癌个人史或家族史的患者。

（20）No information of side effects is provided.

没有提供副作用信息。

（21）These are not all the possible side effects of... For more information, ask your doctor or pharmacist.

这些并不是……的所有可能出现的副作用。有关详细信息，请咨询您的医生或药剂师。

2. 示例

【例 1】

The most frequently reported adverse reactions, from clinical trials of all formulations, all dosages, all drug-therapy durations, and for all indications of ciprofloxacin therapy were nausea (2.5%), diarrhea (1.6%), liver function tests abnormal (1.3%), vomiting (1%), and rash (1%).

在所有制剂、所有剂量、所有药物治疗持续时间，以及所有环丙沙星治疗的适应症的临床试验中，最常报告的不良反应是恶心（2.5%）、腹泻（1.6%）、肝功能异常（1.3%）、呕吐（1%）和皮疹（1%）。

【例 2】

Zyrtec-D may cause serious side effects including fast, pounding, or uneven heartbeats, weakness, tremors, severe restless feeling, hyperactivity, extreme feeling of fear or confusion, vision problems, little or no urinating, severe headache, buzzing in your ears, chest pain, and shortness of breath.

Get medical help right away, if you have any of the symptoms listed above.

The most common side effects of Zyrtec-D include: dizziness, drowsiness, tired feeling, sleep problems (insomnia), dry mouth, nausea, stomach pain, constipation, and trouble concentrating.

塞舒优可能会导致严重的副作用，包括心跳加快、心跳剧烈或心跳不均，虚弱无力，震颤，焦急不安，多动症，极度恐惧或困惑感，视力问题，排尿很少或不排尿，严重的头痛，耳鸣，胸痛和气促。

如果出现上述任何症状，请立即就医。

塞舒优最常见的副作用包括：头晕、嗜睡、疲倦感、睡眠问题（失眠）、口干、恶心、胃痛、便秘、注意力不集中。

5.2.7 禁忌（Contraindications）

禁忌与适应症相反，是指某种药物或该药物中的某些成份在应用于患某些疾病或特殊人群时会产生的不良后果。药品说明书中的“禁忌”一项应列出禁止应用该药品的人群或者疾病的情况。其中包括：“并发症或同时存在的生理状态所致的禁用；人口统计学风险因素所致的禁用；药物只在限定患者亚群使用而因药物风险决不允许药物在更大的亚群中使用；联合用药危险所致的禁用；已观察到严重过敏反应的禁用；因药品中的某些辅料的存在而产生的任何禁忌。”

在药品说明书中，“禁忌”一项表明了此药在何种环境下禁止使用，其包含的禁忌方面的内容需要随着药品使用反馈而及时确认和更新。美国食品药品监督管理局于

2011 年发布了人用处方药和生物制品标签的警告和注意事项、禁忌和黑框警告部分之内容和格式行业指南，指南指出："如果药物没有已知的禁忌，本节必须说明：无。"（If there are no known contraindications for a drug, this section must state: None.）同样，"禁忌"一项中也不包括药物不良反应和慎用的内容。

1. 常用表达

1）词汇

geriatric 老年人　　pregnant woman 孕妇

lactation 哺乳期　　in pregnancy 妊娠期

neonate 新生儿　　infant 婴幼儿

children under... years of age ……岁以下儿童

the first trimester of pregnancy 妊娠期的最初三个月

2）句型

（1）... is contraindicated in patients with...

……患者禁用……

（2）The contraindications are...

禁忌症是……

（3）... be contraindicated in/for...

……对……禁忌

（4）... be allergic/hypersensitive to...

……对……过敏的

（5）... are forbidden to use...

……禁止用……

（6）... must not be administered/given to...

对……不得用……

（7）... should not be used in...

……不得用于……

（8）... be not recommended for...

……不推荐用于……

（9）It is advisable to avoid the use of...

建议避免用于……

2. 示例

【例 1】

Terbinafine Hydrochloride Oral Granules is contraindicated in individuals with a history of allergic reaction to oral terbinafine because of the risk of anaphylaxis.

因存在过敏反应的风险，盐酸特比萘芬口服颗粒剂禁用于对口服特比萘芬有过敏反应史的个体。

【例 2】

Terbinafine Hydrochloride should not be taken by anyone who has problems with his or her liver or kidneys, or by pregnant or nursing women, unless directed by your doctor.

除非医生指示，盐酸特比萘芬不能应用于任何有肝脏或肾脏问题的人群、孕妇、哺乳期女性。

【例 3】

Albendazole Tablets is contraindicated in patients with known hypersensitivity to the benzimidazole class of compounds.

对苯并咪唑类化合物过敏的患者禁用阿苯达唑片。

【例 4】

Patients who are hypersensitive to other NSAIDs are forbidden to use.

对其他非甾体抗炎药过敏者禁用。

【例 5】

Patients with active peptic ulcer are forbidden to use.

活动性消化道溃疡患者禁用。

【例 6】

Children under 12 years of age should not be treated with...

12 岁以下儿童禁用……

【例 7】

Do not administer... to anyone with a history of severe allergic reactions to any component of the vaccine.

不要给任何对疫苗任何成份有严重过敏反应史的人接种……

【例 8】

Oseltamivir is contraindicated in patients with known serious hypersensitivity to oseltamivir or any component of the product. Severe allergic reactions have included anaphylaxis and serious skin reactions.

已知对奥司他韦或该产品的任何成份严重过敏的患者禁用奥司他韦。严重过敏反应包括过敏反应及严重皮肤反应。

【例 9】

Since Lactulose for oral solution contains galactose, it is contraindicated in patients who require a low-galactose diet.

由于口服乳果糖溶液含有半乳糖，因此需要低半乳糖饮食的患者禁用此药。

【例 10】

Do not administer... intrathecally. Inadvertent intrathecal administration may cause death, convulsions, cerebral hemorrhage, coma, paralysis, hyperthermia...

不要鞘内给药……。不慎鞘内给药可能导致死亡、抽搐、脑出血、昏迷、瘫痪、高热……

【例 11】

... is contraindicated in patients who have had an organ transplant or are taking medicine to reduce organ rejection.

……禁用于接受过器官移植或正在服用减少器官排斥反应药物的患者。

【例 12】

In clinical trials, atomoxetine HCL use was associated with an increased risk of mydriasis. It is not recommended for patients with narrow-angle glaucoma.

在临床试验中，托莫西汀的使用会增加散瞳的风险。不建议窄角型青光眼患者使用此药。

5.2.8　注意事项（Precautions）

与“禁忌”一项不同，药品说明书中的“注意事项”一栏列出的是该药品在使用时需要注意的问题。这些问题包括针对不同人群（如孕妇、婴幼儿）的用药说明、药品慎用的情况、用药超过剂量后的应急措施、影响药品药效的因素、用药后需要观察的情况、用药时发生严重不良反应后的治疗方案、临床上体现的重大不良反应、药物的相互作用、评估药物安全性的资料等。在某些药品说明书中，“注意事项”一栏的内容有时会与“警告语”和“用法用量”两部分内容有所重叠。

1. 常用表达

precaution 注意事项

special precaution 特别注意事项

important for the patients 患者须知

renal/kidney function 肾功能

liver/hepatic function 肝功能

blood count 血细胞计数

clotting time 凝血时间

serum concentration 血清浓度

creatinine clearance 肌酸酐清除

specific population 特定人群

blood concentration 血液浓度

serum creatinine test 血清肌酸酐检测

blood pressure 血压

2. 示例

【例 1】

Do not allow the gel to come into contact with the eyes or mucous membranes.

避免凝胶接触眼睛或黏膜。

【例 2】

Stop using... immediately if you experience any skin reactions.

如出现任何皮肤反应，请立即停止使用……

【例 3】

Do not use... on skin breakages or infectious wounds.

……不得用于皮肤破损处及感染性创口。

【例 4】

Do not use the product if you are hypersensitive to...

对……过敏者禁用该产品。

【例 5】

The product should be used with caution in patients with allergic predisposition.

过敏体质者慎用该产品。

【例 6】

The product should be used with caution during pregnancy and breast-feeding.

孕妇、哺乳期女性慎用该产品。

【例 7】

Keep all medications out of the reach of children.

将所有药品置于儿童接触不到的地方。

【例 8】

The use of this product is prohibited when its characteristics change.

本产品性状发生改变时，禁止使用。

【例 9】

Adult supervision is required if it will be used on children.

如果将其用于儿童，则需要成人监督。

【例 10】

Please consult your doctor or pharmacist if you are using other pharmaceutical products.

如果正在使用其他药品，请咨询医生或药师。

【例 11】

If your symptoms persist after three days, please consult your doctor.

治疗三天后不见好转，请咨询医师。

【例 13】

For external use only.

仅供外用。

5.2.9 药物相互作用（Interactions of Drugs）

药物相互作用是指患者在使用一种药物的同时或在一定时间内先后使用另一种药物、食品添加剂或某些食品后出现的复合效应。药物体内相互作用方式包括药动学相互作用和药效学相互作用。我国的《化学药品及生物制品说明书通用格式和撰写指南》指出，“药物相互作用”一栏应“列出与该药产生相互作用的药物或者药物类别，并说明相互作用的结果及合并用药的注意事项”。美国食品药品监督管理局处方药说明书对于“药物相互作用”一栏的主要要求为：“本节必须包含对与其他处方药或非处方药、药物类别或食物，如膳食补充剂、葡萄柚汁，观察或观测到的具有临床意义的相互作用的描述，以及预防或管理这些相互作用的具体的实用说明。如果已知其相互作用的机制，则必须对其进行简要描述。”[This section must contain a description of clinically significant interactions, either observed or predicted, with other prescription or over-the-counter drugs, classes of drugs, or foods (e.g., dietary supplements, grapefruit juice), and specific practical instructions for preventing or managing them. The mechanism(s) of the interaction, if known, must be briefly described.]

示例

【例 1】

Ask a doctor or pharmacist before use if you are taking sedatives or tranquilizers.

如果你正在服用安眠药或镇静剂，请在使用前咨询医生或药师。

【例 2】

Tetracycline may antagonize the bactericidal effect of penicillin and concurrent use of these drugs should be avoided.

四环素可以拮抗青霉素的杀菌作用，应避免同时使用。

【例 3】

There is a risk of ototoxic effects if cisplatin and furosemide tablets are given concomitantly.

如果顺铂和呋塞米同时给药，则存在耳毒性作用的风险。

【例 4】

Furosemide tablets may decrease arterial responsiveness to norepinephrine.

呋塞米片剂可能会降低动脉对去甲肾上腺素的反应性。

【例 5】

The concomitant use of albuterol sulfate syrup and other oral sympathomimetic agents is not recommended since such combined use may lead to cardiovascular effects.

不推荐同时使用硫酸沙丁胺醇糖浆和其他口服拟交感神经药，因为几种药物一起使用可能会对心血管造成影响。

【例 6】

Phenobarbital appears to interfere with the absorption of orally administered griseofulvin, thus decreasing its blood level.

苯巴比妥似乎会干扰口服灰黄霉素的吸收，从而降低其血液浓度。

【例 7】

Heavy alcohol intake for longer than two weeks may produce malabsorption of vitamin B12.

大量饮酒超过两周有可能导致维生素 B12 吸收不良。

【例 8】

Aspirin may increase the serum glucose-lowering action of insulin leading to hypoglycemia.

阿司匹林可能会增加胰岛素的降血糖作用，从而导致低血糖。

【例 9】

No information provided.

尚无相关信息。

【例 10】

Inactivated influenza vaccine can be administered at any time relative to use of oseltamivir phosphate.

灭活流感疫苗可在使用磷酸奥司他韦期间的任何时间接种。

【例 11】

The concomitant use of opioids with other drugs that affect the serotonergic neurotransmitter system has resulted in serotonin syndrome.

阿片类药物与影响血清素能神经递质系统的其他药物同时使用会导致血清素综合征。

5.2.10 贮藏及包装（Storage and Package）

为保证药品的质量，使药品在使用期限内不会因为保存不善而变质，药品说明书中对于"贮藏"及"包装"两项有着严格的要求。我国于 2022 年颁布的《化学药品及生物制品说明书通用格式和撰写指南》中明确规定："贮藏"一项具体条件的表示方法按《中国药典》要求书写，并注明具体温度，如阴凉处（不超过 20℃）保存。生物制品应当同时注明制品保存和运输的环境条件，特别应明确具体温度。"包装"一项包括直接接触药品的包装材料和容器及包装规格，并按该顺序表述。

1. 常用表达

in a cool place 阴凉处

in a dark place 阴暗处

in a dry place 干燥处

room temperature 常 / 室温

cryopreservation 冷藏

away from children 远离儿童

protect from light 避光

protect from heat 避免受热

prevent moisture 防潮

oxidation 氧化

moisture absorption 吸潮

agglomeration 结块

seal 密封

stability 稳定性

validity 有效期

expiration date 失效期

storage life 贮存期限

shelf life 保存期

pack/packing/package 包装

packing for hospital 医院用包装

method of supply 供应方式

package quantity 包装量

ampoule 安瓿

blister pack/package 泡壳包装

bottle 瓶

box 盒

carton 纸盒

can 罐

tube 管

strip 条

sheet 片

vial 小瓶

Cyclo Olefin Polymer vial COP/ 环烯烃药用聚合体小瓶

polyvinylchloride bag PVC/ 聚氯乙烯袋

NDC (National Drug Code) 国家药品验证号

2. 示例

【例 1】

Please keep all medicines out of the reach of children.

请将所有药品放在儿童接触不到的地方。

【例 2】

Please store capsules and tablets at room temperature between 15℃ to 25℃.

请在 15 ~ 25 摄氏度的室温下储存胶囊和片剂。

【例 3】

Please keep tablets in the light resistant container that it comes in.

请将片剂保存在随附的耐光容器中。

【例 4】

Please store oral suspension at room temperature between 15 ℃ to 30 ℃, for up to 60 days. You can also store oral suspension in the refrigerator between 1℃ to 5℃. Do not freeze.

请将口服混悬液储存在 15 ~ 30 摄氏度的室温下，存储时间最长可达 60 天；也可以将其储存在 1 ~ 5 摄氏度的冰箱中。请勿冷冻。

【例 5】

Do not use... after the expiration date on the bottle.

请勿在瓶上标注的有效期后使用……。

【例 6】

Protect from light. Keep covered in carton until ready to use. Store upright at controlled room temperature 15℃ to 30℃. Protect from freezing.

避光。使用前，请将药品置于盒中储存。请在 15 ~ 30 摄氏度的室温下直立存放药品。谨防冷冻。

【例 7】

If unable to use within this time period, the reconstituted solution can be stored under refrigeration (2℃–8℃) for up to 2 hours in the 50 mL labeled syringe.

如果在这段时间内无法使用，可将复原溶液在 50 毫升容量的注射器中冷藏（2 ~ 8 摄氏度）最长两个小时。

【例 8】

The solution will keep for three years if stored at a temperature below 4℃.

此溶液可在 4 摄氏度以下保存三年。

【例 9】

Store at 15℃ –20℃. Keep dry and foil intact.

储存温度在 15 ~ 20 摄氏度。保持干燥，箔纸完好。

【例 10】

Capsules: Store at room temperature; avoid excessive heat; keep tightly closed.

胶囊：室温储存；避免过热；盖严。

【例 11】

Store at room temperature; discard unused portion after 7 days if kept at room temperature or after 14 days if refrigerated; keep bottles tightly closed.

室温储存，室温储存 7 天或冷藏储存 14 天后需丢弃尚未使用的药品，紧闭瓶口。

【例 12】

Store the dry powder below 30℃.

在 30 摄氏度以下保存干粉。

【例 13】

Presentation 15 capsules.

15 粒胶囊包装。

【例 14】

Packages: Box containing one 60 mg bottle.

包装：盒装，每盒 1 瓶，每瓶 60 毫克。

【例 15】

Packages: Foil sealed, 65 mg tablets (20 tablets).

包装：箔密封的 65 毫克片剂（共 20 片）。

【例 16】

Package: 5 mg vial (box of 6).

包装：5 毫克小瓶装（6 盒装）。

【例 17】

Packing bottle of 60 capsules 250 mg. Box of 12 capsules 250 mg in blister.

瓶装：每瓶 60 粒胶囊，每粒含量 250 毫克。盒装：每盒 12 粒胶囊，每粒含量 250 毫克。

【例 18】

Bottle for pediatric use: 10 mg granule contains 0.5 mg ampicillin.

瓶装儿童用颗粒剂：10 毫克颗粒剂含有 0.5 毫克氨苄青霉素。

【例 19】

Packing bottle of 60 sugar coated tablets for pediatric use.

瓶装：每瓶 60 片糖衣片，供儿童服用。

【例 20】

Packing materials: Aluminum tube; Packing size: 10 g/tube.

包装材料：铝管；包装规格：10 克 / 管。

【例 21】

Mode of issue: Medicine A is issued in vials containing 2.4 g of penicillin.

包装方式：药物 A 小瓶包装，内有 2.4 克青霉素。

【例 22】

Paint in glass bottles of 30 mL.

玻璃瓶装涂剂，每瓶 30 毫升。

【例 23】

Each canister provides 200 sprays.

每罐可喷 200 次。

【例 24】

Penicillin G potassium for injection is available in the following package sizes: 10 vials per carton, each 1 vial contains 5,000,000 units. Each million unit contains approximately 6.8 milligrams of sodium and 65.6 milligrams of potassium.

注射用青霉素 G 钾包装规格如下：每箱 10 瓶，每瓶 500 万单位。每百万单位含有大约 6.8 毫克钠和 65.6 毫克钾。

5.2.11 其他信息（Other Information）

除上述基本信息外，药品说明书还标注了一些有助于患者了解药品相关信息、更好使用药品的事项，如有效期（Shelf Life）、执行标准（Specifications）、药品批准文号（Drug Approval No.）、说明书修订日期（Revision Date）、药品上市许可持有人（Marketing Authorization Holder）、生产企业（Manufacturer）等。

Exercises

Exercise I　Translate the following into English.

1. 低血糖是一种与胰岛素相关的、常见的不良反应。严重低血糖会引发癫痫，甚至导致死亡。（hypoglycemia/seizures）
2. 继续摄入足量的钙，但不要摄入过量的钙。（calcium）
3. 处方和非处方药的滥用指的是将药物用于医生处方之外的目的或方式。（prescription/nonprescription）
4. 心绞痛被描述为一种严重的心脏病。（angina）
5. 尚不清楚无菌水对儿童是否安全有效。（sterile water）

Exercise II　Translate the following into Chinese.

1. Penicillin is active against a number of types of bacteria including streptococcus pneumoniae, listeria, peptostreptococcus.
2. Cefaclor is indicated in the treatment of the infections when caused by susceptible strains of the microorganisms.
3. In patients with normal renal function, chronic hypocalcaemia may be associated with an increase in serum creatinine.
4. A drug interaction can be defined as an interaction between a drug and another substance that prevents the drug from performing as expected.
5. The main ingredient of this product is a compound preparation, and its components are: licorice extract powder 112.5 mg, opioid powder 4 mg, camphor 2 mg, star anise oil 2 mg, and sodium benzoate 2 mg.

Exercise III　Fill in the blanks of a package insert of a drug based on the information given.

Aspirin is a medicine used to reduce the risk of having a heart attack in people who have heart disease or to reduce the risk of stroke in people who have had a stroke before.

Aspirin may cause ____________________ (严重的副作用) including: ringing in your ears, confusion, hallucinations, rapid breathing, seizure, ____________________ (严重恶心), ____________________ (呕吐), ____________________ (胃痛).

____________________ (剂量):

Adults and children 12 years and over: ____________________ (4 小时 1 片), not to exceed 12 tablets in 24 hours.

Children under 12 years: ____________________ (咨询医生).

Packaging:

Tablets and caplets are available in the following package types:

Travel pack—12 tablets;

Bottles of 50, 100, 200, and 400 tablets.

Drug Interactions:

____________________ (尚无提供信息).

Patients Information:

If ____________________ (怀孕或哺乳), ask a health professional before use.

____________________ (放在儿童接触不到的地方). In case of overdose, get medical help right away.

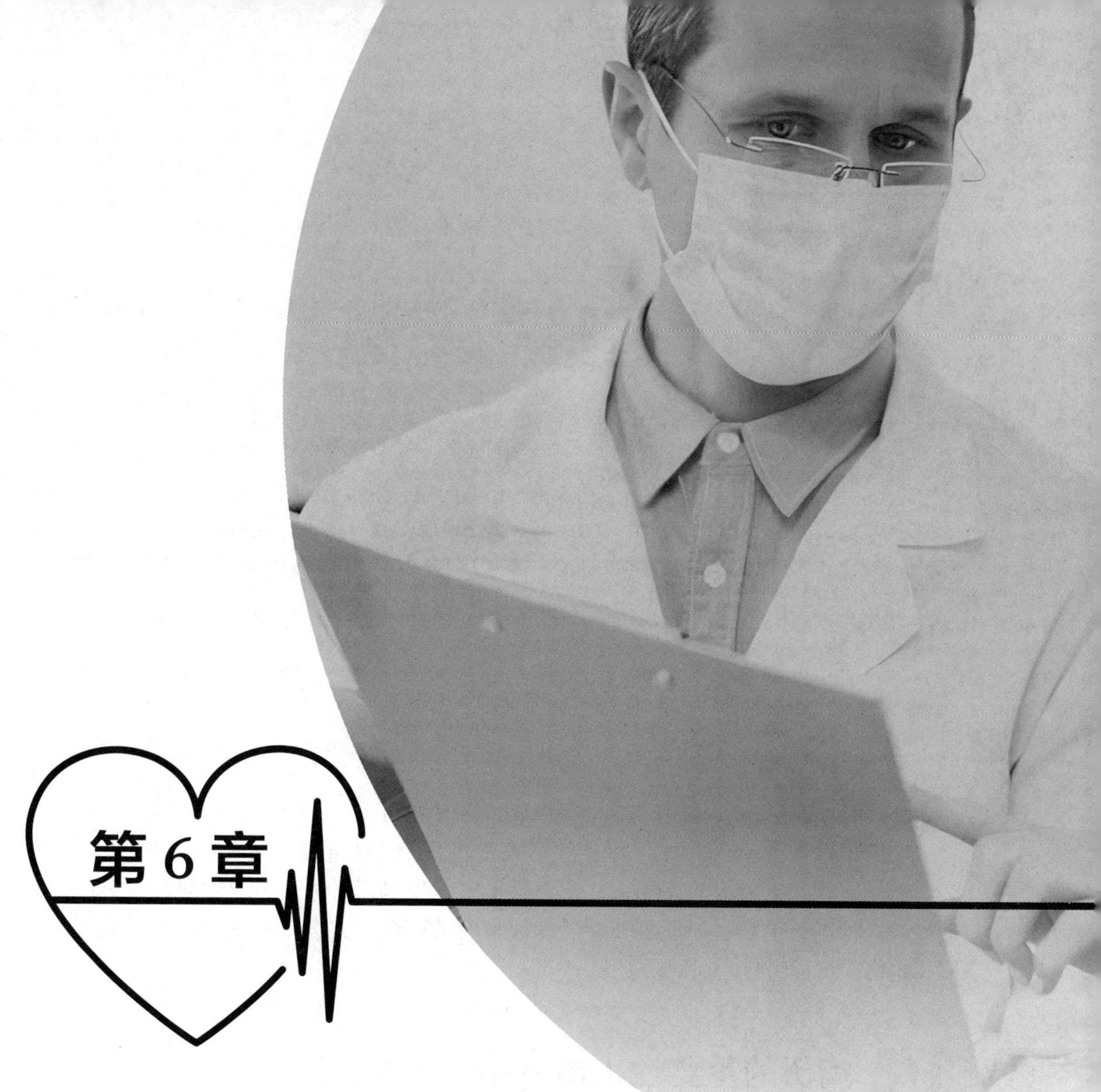

第 6 章

病　历
（Case History）

Medicines are not meant to live on.

不能靠药物度日。

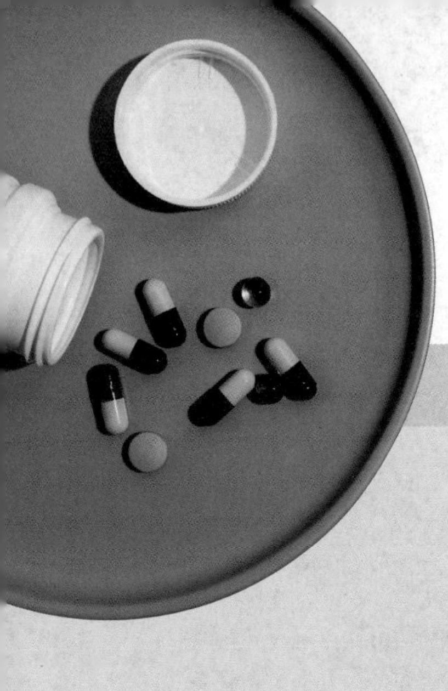

Warm-up

1. If you're a doctor, what will you want to know from a patient when you write a disease history?
2. Please list some elements which would help you communicate with the patients, say, friendly behavior, neat dress, good manners, and other effective communication skills.

病历（Case History, CH）是指医务人员在医疗活动过程中形成的文字、符号、图表、影像、切片等资料的总和。它记录整个医疗案例，医务人员通过问诊、查体、辅助检查、诊断、治疗、护理等医疗活动获得有关资料，并进行归纳、分析、整理，按照规定格式形成医疗活动记录。

6.1 病历的重要性（Importance of CH）

病历是医疗从业人员做出准确诊断的基础，它为医疗、教学与科研提供了重要的基本资料。病历可作为健康保健档案和医疗保险的依据，同时也是涉及医疗纠纷和诉讼的重要依据。病历的写作是医生的基本功，可作为考核其临床实际工作能力、评价医疗质量和学术水平的内容。

6.2 病历写作的基本要求（Basic Requirements of Writing CH）

病历要求客观、真实、准确、及时、完整地记录患者病情和诊疗经过。我国卫生部要求2010年3月1日起，在全国各医疗机构施行修订完善后的《病历书写基本规范》。该规范对各医疗机构的病历书写行为进行了详细规定，以保证病历质量，保障医疗质量和安全，主要有以下要求：

（1）病历书写应规范使用医学术语，文字工整，字迹清晰，表述准确，语句通顺，标点正确。

（2）病历书写应当使用蓝黑墨水、碳素墨水，需复写的病历资料可以使用蓝或黑色油水的圆珠笔。计算机打印的病历应当符合病历保存的要求。

（3）病历书写过程中出现错字时，应当用双线画在错字上，保留原记录清楚、可辨，并注明修改时间、修改人签名。不得采用刮、粘、涂等方法掩盖或去除原来的字迹。

（4）病历应当按照规定的内容书写，并由相应医务人员签名。上级医务人员有审查修改下级医务人员书写的病历的责任。

（5）病历书写一律使用阿拉伯数字书写日期和时间，采用 24 小时制记录。

（6）对需取得患者书面同意方可进行的医疗活动，应当由患者本人签署知情同意书。患者不具备完全民事行为能力时，应当由其法定代理人签字；患者因病无法签字时，应当由其授权的人员签字；为抢救患者，在法定代理人或被授权人无法及时签字的情况下，可由医疗机构负责人或者授权的负责人签字。

因实施保护性医疗措施不宜向患者说明情况的，应当将有关情况告知患者近亲属，由患者近亲属签署知情同意书，并及时记录。患者无近亲属或者近亲属无法签署知情同意书的，由患者的法定代理人或者关系人签署同意书。

6.3 病历的分类（Classification of CH）

病历包括门（急）诊病历和住院病历。门（急）诊病历是为了记录在门诊或急诊就诊的患者的相关医疗情况，应当由接诊医师在患者就诊时及时完成，较为简洁明了，只描述重点。一般的门诊病历书写内容包括：就诊时间（Time）、科别（Department）、一般资料（General Data / G.D.）、主诉（Chief Complaint / C.C.）、现病史（Present Illness / P.I.）、体格检查（Physical Examination / P.E.）、初步诊断（Tentative Diagnosis 或 Impression/Imp.）及治疗意见（Treatment 或 Response/Rp.）和医生签名（Signature）。

住院病历是指患者入院后，由经治医师通过问诊、查体、辅助检查获得有关资料，并对这些资料归纳分析书写而成的完整记录。在诊疗过程中，它还包含病程记录（指继入院记录后对患者病情和诊疗过程所进行的连续性记录，包括患者的病情变化情况、重要的辅助检查结果及临床意义、上级医师查房意见、会诊意见、医师分析讨论意见、所采取的诊疗措施及效果、医嘱更改及理由、向患者及其近亲属告知的重要事项等），即自入院至出院整个过程的记录。

目前，国内外对病历的书写都没有统一、固定的格式，具体格式因医院而异，因人而异。病历记录的项目和内容也简繁不一，但基本内容大致相同。本章参照国内外多种病历的格式，重点介绍住院病历的基本内容和写法。

6.4 住院病历（CH of Inpatients）

住院病历的主要项目有：

（1）一般资料（General Data）；

（2）主诉（Chief Complaint）；

（3）现病史（Present Illness）；

（4）既往病史（Past History）；

（5）个人史（Personal History）；

（6）家族史（Family History）；

（7）系统回顾（System Review）；

（8）体格检查（Physical Examination）；

（9）实验室数据（Laboratory Data）；

（10）病史小结 / 病历摘要（History Summary）；

（11）诊断 / 印象（Diagnosis/Impression）；

（12）治疗（Treatment）；

（13）病程记录（Progress Note）；

（14）出院小结（Discharge Summary）。

在具体的病历写作中，我们可根据实际情况合并或删减项目。

6.4.1 一般资料 (General Data)

1. 内容和要求

一般资料即患者的基本信息（Personal Information / Biographical Data），也可被称为患者身份（Identification），主要包括：病历号（Case No.）；姓名（Name）；性别（Sex），应填写"男"（Male）或者"女"（Female）；年龄（Age）；民族或国籍（Nationality）；出生日期（Date of Birth）；出生地（Place of Birth）；身份证号码（ID No.）；婚姻状况（Marital Status），一般填写"单身"（Single/Unmarried）、"已婚"（Married）或者"离婚"（Divorced）；职业（Occupation）；住址及电话（Address and Phone No.），英文住址按照从小到大的顺序书写；邮编（Post Code）；病史可靠程度（Reliability），一般填写"可靠"（Reliable）、"不可靠"（Unreliable）、"不完全可靠"（Not Entirely）、"混乱"（Confused）或者"无法获得"（Unobtainable）；病史提供者（Complainer of History），一般可填写"患者本人"（Patient Himself/Herself）、"患者丈夫"（Patient's Husband）、"患儿母亲"（Patient's Mother）、"交警"（Traffic Police）等；入院时病情（Patient Condition），可填写"稳定"（Stable）、"不稳定"（Unstable）、"相对稳定"（Relative Stable）、"危重"（Critical）等；入院日期

（Date of Admission）；记录时间（Date of Record）等。

一般资料的项目往往是按照固定格式印刷在医院病历首页上，内容可由患者或接诊的医护人员根据具体情况填写。

2. 示例

Case No.: 409867

Name: Zhang Qingmei **Sex：** Female

Age: 42 years old **Date of Birth：** 6–19–1980

Marital Status: Married **Place of Birth:** Dalian, Liaoning

Occupation: Housekeeper **ID No.:** XXX

Residence and Phone No.: Building 5, No. 3 Yichun Road, Dalian 13XXX

Reliability: Reliable **Complainer of History:** Patient herself

Patient Condition: Stable **Date of Admission:** 3–22–2023

Date of Record: 3–22–2023

6.4.2 主诉（Chief Complaints）

1. 内容和要求

主诉是客观记录患者自己所诉说的疾病症状或就诊的主要原因，包括就诊时间、发病时间、持续时间等。这部分须精炼准确，有高度的概括性，多用省略句、短语或短句，不使用人物称谓和 a、the 等冠词。

例如，患者“主诉饭后半小时感到下腹痛”，可记录为“C.C. lower abdominal pain half an hour after eating”；主诉“Patient has had sore throat for three days”可简写为“Sore throat for three days”；“一两个月以来，工作时就感觉呼吸困难和眩晕”，可简写为“For 1 or 2 months, dyspnea and dizziness on work”。

住院病历的主诉部分多用省略句，有时也会用完整句。叙述的主要症状一般不超过三个，各个症状应陈述清楚其各自持续的时间。患者描述过去出现的症状都用过去时，如果是在过去持续一段时间的症状，要用过去进行时。如果患者的症状是从过去某一时间一直持续到现在，可用现在完成时。

2. 常用表达

1）表示症状及持续时间

（1）症状 + for + 时间

cough for 2 days 咳嗽两天

（2）症状 + of + 时间 + duration

nausea and dizziness of three days' duration 恶心眩晕三天

（3）症状 + 时间 + in duration

a headache with nausea one month in duration 头痛伴恶心一个月

（4）时间 + of + 症状

two-day history of fever 发热两天

（5）症状 + since + 时间

low fever and coughing since last weekend 自上周末发低烧、咳嗽

2）表示患者就诊或入院及原因

（1）present / appear / complain of

The patient presented severe diarrhea for two days.

患者就诊时严重腹泻两日。

（2）be admitted because of

The 55-year-old female was admitted because of subcostal pain for three days.

55 岁女性，因肋下疼痛三天入院。

（3）suffer from

The patient suffered from chest pain while walking up the stairs.

患者上楼梯时感到胸痛。

（4）enter... with complaints of

The patient entered the emergency room with complaints of palpitation and dyspnea following physical exertion.

患者入急诊室，主诉剧烈体力活动后心悸和呼吸困难。

（5）be referred to... because of / due to

The patient was referred to our clinic due to suspected anterior encephalocele.

患者因怀疑前部的脑膨出来我处就诊。

3. 示例

【例 1】

Palpitations for more than two years, and chills, fever, dyspnea and edema of the ankle for half a month.

心悸两年余，近半月来寒战、发热、呼吸困难及脚踝水肿。

【例 2】

Night sweat, coughing severe at night, easily agitated, increasing abdominal pain.

盗汗、夜间咳嗽剧烈、烦躁、腹痛加剧。

【例 3】

A 60-year-old male with a history of ulcerative colitis complains of four months of worsening back stiffness, three weeks of a sore on the leg and two days of fevers and bloody, painless diarrhea.

60 岁男性，有溃疡性结肠炎病史，主诉为背部僵硬加重四个月，腿痛三周，发热和带血、无痛腹泻两天。

【例 4】

This patient presented today complaining of burning pain when bending two hours after eating. She indicated the problem location was the stomach upper left locally and severity of condition was worsening.

患者今日就诊，主诉进食两小时后弯腰时胃左上方局部灼痛，疼痛加剧。

6.4.3 现病史（Present Illness）

1. 内容和要求

现病史是对主诉的进一步延伸，主要应从医生的角度，记载当前疾病的发生时间、经过、发病方式、可能病因与诱因、严重程度、发作频率、进展情况、治疗情况等。现病史应完整有序地记录病史的信息，但并不需要分析和解释病史。

这部分内容应尽量使用完整的语句，多用陈述句。描述起病及就诊情况用一般过去时，记录患者现在的情况或一般情况用现在时，强调“疾病一直持续到现在”用现在完成时，表示“以前有过但现在未再出现的症状或疾病”则用过去完成时。

2. 常用表达

1）表示“感觉 / 有……症状”

start/begin having/feeling/presenting 开始有 / 感觉 / 呈现症状

suffer from 遭受

have an attack of 病情发作

complain that/of 主诉

notice/perceive the onset of 注意到 / 觉察到……的开始

She started feeling dull pain in the lower abdomen last week.

她从上周开始感到下腹隐隐作痛。

The patient first noticed the onset of cramp on Friday.

患者在星期五第一次注意到抽筋。

2）表示“与……有关 / 无关”

be associated with 与……有关

have/make relation to 与……有关

have/make no relation to 与……无关

have correlation with 与……有关

correlate with 与……相关

It can be associated with raised blood pressure.

这可能与血压升高有关

Doctors attempted to correlate symptoms with defective development.

医生试图将症状与发育缺陷联系起来。

3）表示病情变化

（1）在……情况下加重 / 减轻

become worse/exacerbated/aggravated after taking meals 饭后加重

be relieved/alleviated by standing up 站立后缓解

become more severe with breathing and cough 随呼吸和咳嗽而加重

（2）症状好转

feel better than before 感觉比以前好

take a favorable turn 好转

take a turn for the better 好转

improve 好转

make favorable progress 好转

turn/change for the better 好转

be better 好转

（3）症状消失

disappear 消失

subside 消退

regress 消退

clear up 消失

vanish 消失

dissolve 消失

die/fade away 消失

（4）症状时好时坏

wane and wax 时强时弱

hang in the balance 安危未定

4）表示体温或血压升降

rise / go up to 升至

have risen / gone up to 已升至

go up from... to 从……升至

be elevated to 升至

fall/decline/abate abruptly 迅速下降

sudden drop/elevation　骤降 / 升

fall/elevate gradually 渐降 / 升

fall/elevate from... to 由……降 / 升至

be/become lower day by day　一天天下降

drop / be reduced to normal 降至正常

have gone down / dropped to 已降至

return/revert to normal 回复到正常

maintain/stabilize at a level of 维持 / 稳定在……水平

fever disappeared 热退了

do not go up over / exceed 不超过

fluctuate/vary between... and 在……与……之间波动

range from... to 在……至……范围内

an average temperature of 38.5℃ 平均体温为 38.5 摄氏度

have a fever / a temperature of 39.2℃ 体温为 39.2 摄氏度

3. 示例

【例 1】

P.I.: The patient felt upper abdominal pain two days ago and didn't pay enough attention to it because the pain was not severe. At 7 o'clock this morning, he fainted suddenly and rejected fresh blood and gore. Then hemafecia began. He was then rushed to the hospital. The patient was accepted and received emergent treatment for upper gastrointestinal bleeding and hemorrhagic shock.

现病史：两天前，患者自觉上腹疼痛，因较轻微并未在意。今晨七点突然昏倒，有新鲜血液和血块呕出，并便血，后被紧急送往医院，以“上消化道出血并失血性休克”入院急诊治疗。

【例 2】

Ms. J. K. is an 83-year-old retired nurse with a long history of hypertension that was previously well controlled on diuretic therapy.

She was well until 11 p.m. on the night prior to admission when she noted the onset of "aching pain under her breast bone" while sitting, watching television. The pain was described as "heavy" and "toothache" like. It was not noted to radiate, nor increase with exertion. She denied nausea, vomiting, diaphoresis, palpitations, dizziness, or loss of consciousness. She took two tablespoons of antacid without relief, but did manage to fall asleep. In the morning she awoke free of pain, however upon walking to the bathroom, the pain returned with increased severity. At this time, she called her daughter, who gave her an aspirin and brought her immediately to the emergency room.

Aside from hypertension and her postmenopausal state, the patient denies other coronary artery disease risk factors, such as diabetes, cigarette smoking, hypercholesterolemia or family history for heart disease.

J. K. 女士是一名 83 岁的退休护士，有长期高血压病史，此前通过利尿剂治疗得到了很好的控制。

入院前的晚上 11 点，她发现自己坐着看电视时“胸骨下隐隐作痛”。疼痛被描述为“很重”和“牙痛”一样。没有注意到辐射痛，也没有随着运动而加重。她否认恶心、呕吐、出汗、心悸、头晕或失去意识。服用了两汤匙抗酸剂，没有缓解症状，但还是睡着了。早上醒来时，她没有疼痛，但是当她去洗手间时，疼痛加重。这时，她给女儿打了电话，女儿让她服用了一片阿司匹林，并立即带她去了急诊室。

除高血压和绝经后状态外，患者否认其他冠状动脉疾病的危险因素，如糖尿病、吸烟、高胆固醇血症或心脏病家族史。

6.4.4 既往史（Past History）

1. 内容和要求

既往史又称过去病史，主要记录患者的既往健康状况和过去曾经患过的疾病及治疗等情况。主要内容包括曾患疾病、传染病史、过敏史、主要传染病、外伤、手术、住院情况等，医师均需对其进行详细询问，尤其是与现在疾病相关的，更应该详细记述。记录顺序一般是按照时间顺序先后排列。

如果患者有过敏史，医师可以在这部分用红色或者不同颜色的墨水笔记录下致敏物，也可以在后面单独列在过敏史项目中。

医师在这部分经常用不连贯或者不完整的英语表达，省略句和短语较为常用。动词一般用过去时，但发生在过去某一个时间以前的情况通常用过去完成时。

2. 常用表达

1）表示既往健康状况

health state was good/bad 健康状况佳 / 差

have enjoyed good health until 在……之前一直健康

have been sound/well/healthy until 在……之前一直健康

have suffered from / contracted 曾患

be attacked/troubled by 患

be liable/subject/apt to 易患

tend to 易患

be hospitalized for 因……住院

be admitted into the hospital for 因……住院

be discharged/dismissed from hospital / out of hospital 出院

2）表示有无病史

no history of / no related history of / have no history of 无……史

deny any history of / experiencing 否认……史

have a/no history of allergy to 有 / 无……过敏史

be diagnosed as having 被诊断患有

be inoculated with 接种过

3. 示例

【例 1】

Past medical history: The patient never contracted TB and pneumonia before. He suffered from bronchitis two years ago. Function of the lung was checked normal last year. In 2008, he contracted acute mesenteric arterial occlusion. The circulation system, digestive system, endocrine system, urinary system, and nerve system are normal. No surgery was ever done.

既往病史：患者未感染过肺结核或肺炎，两年前患支气管炎，去年肺功能检查正常。2008 年，患急性肠系膜动脉闭塞。循环系统、消化系统、内分泌系统、泌尿系统和神经系统均正常。未接受过任何手术。

【例 2】

Past Health

General: Relatively good.

Infectious Diseases: Usual childhood illnesses. No history of rheumatic fever.

Immunizations: Flu vaccine yearly.

Allergic to penicillin—developed a diffuse rash after an injection 20 years ago.

Transfusions: 4 units received in 1980 for GI hemorrhage, transfusion complicated by Hepatitis B infection.

Hospitalizations, Operations, Injuries:

(1) Normal childbirth 48 years ago.

(2) 1980 gastrointestinal hemorrhage, see below.

(3) 9/1995 chest pain—see history of present illness.

(4) Last mammogram 1994, flexible sigmoidoscopy 1997.

既往史

总体：比较好。

传染病：常见的儿童疾病。无风湿热病史。

免疫接种：每年接种流感疫苗。

对青霉素过敏——在 20 年前注射后出现弥漫性皮疹。

输血：1980 年，因胃肠道出血接受 4 个单位的输血，输血并发乙型肝炎感染。

住院、手术、受伤：

（1）48 年前，正常分娩。

（2）1980 年，胃肠道出血，见下文。

（3）1995 年 9 月，胸痛——见现病史。

（4）1994 年，最后一次乳房 X 光检查，1997 年柔性乙状结肠镜检查。

6.4.5 个人史（Personal History）

1. 内容和要求

个人史主要记录患者的生活史，包括生活习惯、职业与工作情况、爱好（如吸烟、饮酒）等。如果患者是女性，医生还应记录其婚育和月经情况；如果患者是儿童，还应包括其为自然产或剖腹产、母乳喂养或配方奶喂养、发育、预防接种等情况。

个人史多用陈述句表示，有时也用省略句。个人史陈述既有患者过去的情况，也有现在的习惯，因此谓语动词既可以用一般过去时和过去完成时，也可以用一般现在时或现在完成时。

2. 常用表达

1）表示嗜好

have a long history of smoking/drinking　有很长的吸烟 / 饮酒史

have a like/dislike of/for　喜欢 / 不喜欢

admit to excessive use of　承认过度使用

2）表示职业

work/act/serve as　工作

be engaged in　从事

3）表示婚育、月经史

have been married for... with/without　结婚……生育 / 未曾生育

have history/no history of abortion/premature birth　有 / 无流产 / 早产史

have delivered / have given birth to normal/abnormal　生育过正常 / 非正常

be delivered... before the expected date of childbirth　比预产期提前……出生

have a normal/regular period every... days that last... days 经期正常，周 / 经期……天

3. 示例

【例 1】

Born and grew up in Shandong. No history of excessive alcohol and tobacco use. No drug allergic history. No exposure history to epidemic areas of infectious disease.

在山东出生长大。否认过量饮酒及吸烟史。无药物过敏史。无传染病疫区暴露史。

【例 2】

The ill baby was born by caesarean section. On the whole she has been formula-feeding because her mother has little milk. No teeth have grown out when she is seven months old.

病儿为剖腹产，因母乳少，基本为配方奶喂养，7 个月时无牙齿萌出。

【例 3】

Personal History

(1) Mrs. Johnson is widowed and lives with one of her daughters.

(2) Occupation: She worked as a nurse to age 67; now retired.

(3) Habits: No cigarettes or alcohol. Does not follow any special diet.

(4) Born in South Carolina, came to New York in 1931. She has never been outside of the United States.

(5) Present environment: Lives in a one-bedroom apartment on the third floor of a building with an elevator.

(6) Financial: Receives social security and medicare, and is supported by her children.

(7) Psychosocial: The patient is generally an alert and active woman despite her arthritic symptoms. She understands that she is having a "heart attack" at the present time and she appears to be extremely anxious.

个人史

（1）约翰逊夫人守寡，和一个女儿住在一起。

（2）职业：她当护士到 67 岁，现已退休。

（3）习惯：不抽烟，不喝酒，无任何特殊的饮食习惯。

（4）出生于南卡罗来纳州，1931 年来到纽约，从未离开过美国。

（5）目前环境：住在一个公寓三层的一居室内，有电梯。

（6）经济状况：接受社会保障和医疗保险，且由其子女赡养。

（7）社会心理状况：尽管有关节炎的症状，患者通常是一个敏锐且活跃的女性。她知道自己现在"心脏病发作"了，看起来非常焦虑。

6.4.6 家族史（Family History）

1. 内容和要求

家族史主要记录与患者关系密切的家庭成员（父母、兄弟姊妹、配偶、子女及其他近亲）的健康状况，尤其是传染病和遗传病的相关情况。医师还应特别询问成员是否与患者有同样的疾病，这对于正确诊断患者疾病有着非常重要的意义。如有直系家族成员死亡，患者需说明其死亡原因及时间。

书写家族史可使用完整的句子，也可用省略句。因为该部分涉及患者及家属的过去和现在的情况，谓语动词可用一般现在时、现在进行时和一般过去时。

2. 常用表达

1）家族有 / 无……病

there's a/no family history of 有 / 无……病家族史

no family history of 无……病家族史

2）家族有……倾向

his family history showed/revealed 他的家族史显示

there was a strong family history of 有很强的家族病史

There was a high incidence of... in the family.

家族的……发生率很高。

There is a hereditary tendency to... in the family.

家族遗传倾向于……

3）家族史无异常

Family history was alleged not remarkable.

据说，家族病史并不显著。

Family history was no contributory.

家族病史与此无关。

4）因……而死

death was due to 因……而死

die of/from... at the age of 在……岁时死于……

Death was coincided with the patient's illness.

该患者因病去世。

5）（未）曾接触过……患者

the patient has a/no history of intimate contact with 患者有 / 无……亲密接触史

6）健康 / 不健康

be in good health / healthy / living and well 健康

have a bad health / unhealthy 不健康

3. 示例

【例 1】

Father is living and well. Mother died of lung cancer; a sister of tuberculosis.

父亲体健；母亲死于肺癌，一个姐姐 / 妹妹死于结核病。

【例 2】

His father suffered from chronic stomach disorder and died of duodenal ulcer, no nervous or mental disease, no cancer.

他的父亲有慢性胃部疾病，死于十二指肠溃疡，无神经系统或精神病史，无癌症。

【例 3】

Family History

The patient was brought up by an aunt; her mother died at the age of 36 from kidney failure; her father died at the age of 41 in a car accident. Her husband died 9 years ago of seizures and pneumonia. She had one sister who died in childbirth. She has 4 daughters (ages 65, 60, 56, 48) who are all healthy, and had a son who died at the age of 2 from pneumonia. She has 12 grandchildren, 6 great grandchildren, and 4 great, great grandchildren. There is no known family history of hypertension, diabetes, or cancer.

家族史

患者由阿姨抚养长大；其母在 36 岁时死于肾衰竭；其父在 41 岁时死于一场车祸。丈夫 9 年前死于癫痫和肺炎。一个姐姐死于难产。她有 4 个女儿（65 岁、60 岁、56 岁、48 岁），她们都很健康；一个儿子在 2 岁时死于肺炎。她有 12 个孙子 / 女、6 个曾孙 / 女和 4 个曾曾孙 / 女。没有已知的高血压、糖尿病或癌症家族病史。

6.4.7 系统回顾（System Review）

1. 内容和要求

系统回顾主要记录对各系统疾病与症状的回顾，以期发现与现病症有关的线索和证据。这部分内容虽然不多，但是对进一步评估有很大价值。书写时，医师应避免面面俱到，只记录有价值的症状和体征，其余可省略。这部分常用省略句和短句。

2. 常用表达

- **respiratory system 呼吸系统**

cough 咳嗽
sputum 咳痰
short of breath 呼吸困难
chest pain 胸痛
night sweating 盗汗
fever 发热

- **circulatory system 循环系统**

palpitation 心悸

chest pain 胸痛

hemoptysis 咯血

edema 水肿

syncope 晕厥

dizziness 头晕

- **digestive system 消化系统**

belching 嗳气

sour regurgitation 反酸

abdominal distension 腹胀

abdominal pain 腹痛

diarrhea 腹泻

nausea and vomiting 恶心和呕吐

- **urinary system 泌尿系统**

difficulty in micturition 排尿困难

frequency and urgency of micturition 尿频和尿急

painful micturition 尿痛

- **hematopoietic system 造血系统**

fatigue 乏力

bleeding 出血

- **endocrine system 内分泌系统**

heat intolerance 怕热

excessive sweating 多汗

polydipsia 烦渴

hand tremble 手抖

wasting and obesity 消瘦和肥胖

- **nervous system 神经系统**

headache 头痛

coma 晕厥

vertigo 眩晕

insomnia 失眠

hemiplegia 偏瘫

aphasia 失语

- **motor system 运动系统**

joint pain 关节痛

numbness 麻木

claudication 跛行

paralysis 瘫痪

3. 示例

【例 1】

He denies nausea and vomiting, fever or chills, shortness of breath, cough, chest pain, abdominal pain, or urinary symptoms.

他否认恶心和呕吐、发热或发冷、呼吸急促、咳嗽、胸痛、腹痛或泌尿系统症状。

【例 2】

System Review

Respiratory system: No history of dyspnea, slight chest pain when exerting himself

Circulation system: No history of hypertension or palpitations

Breast: Non-contributory

Digestive system: Bowel movement abnormal for about two months

Urinary system: No history of urinary incontinence or hematuria

Endocrine system: Non-contributory

Nervous system: No history of headache or vertigo

系统回顾

呼吸系统：无呼吸困难，用力时会有轻微胸痛

循环系统：无高血压或心悸

乳房：未查

消化系统：近两月排便异常

泌尿系统：无尿失禁或血尿病史

内分泌系统：未查

神经系统：无头痛或眩晕病史

【例 3】

Muscular: Weakness of muscles

Integumentary: (–) Cyanosis

Respiratory: Tachypnea; (+) DOB, (+) coarse crackles, (+) wheezes

Digestive: Loss of appetite, vomit after ingesting milk

肌肉：肌肉无力

皮肤：无发绀

呼吸（系统）：呼吸急促，DOB（+），粗湿啰音（+），喘鸣（+）

消化（系统）：厌食，摄入牛奶后呕吐

6.4.8 体格检查（Physical Examination）

1. 内容和要求

体格检查是诊断中必不可少的步骤。医生得到相关信息后，在问诊的基础上，通

过视诊（inspection）、听诊（auscultation）、触诊（palpation）和叩诊（percussion）找出与患者疾病有关的体征，以做出正确的诊断，或者进一步支持或否定前面提出的鉴别诊断。体格检查主要包括一般资料、皮肤黏膜、头颈、胸腹、肛门直肠、泌尿生殖、四肢脊柱、神经反射等内容。记录体检结果不一定面面俱到，有些项目只有在需要时才进行，应尽量做到有针对性，有些内容仅记录数据即可。

体格检查的书写也有一定的格式，医师须根据实际要求书写。体检记录常用短语、缩略语或省略句，有时也用陈述句，多用一般现在时，有时也用一般过去时。

2. 示例

【例 1】

Physical Examination

T 103 ℉, P 130/min, R 23/min, BP 100/60 mmHg.

He is well developed and moderately nourished. Active position. His consciousness was not clear. His face was cadaverous and the skin was not stained yellow. No cyanosis. No pigmentation. No skin eruption. Spider angioma was not seen. No pitting edema. Superficial lymph nodes were not found enlarged.

体　检

体温 103 ℉，脉搏 130/ 分钟，呼吸 23/ 分钟，血压 100/60 毫米汞柱。

发育良好，营养适中。自主体位。意识不清，面色苍白，皮肤无黄染。无发绀。无色素沉着。无皮疹。未看到蜘蛛痔。无可凹性水肿。浅表淋巴结未见肿大。

【例 2】

Heart

No bulge and no abnormal impulse or thrills in the precordial area. The point of maximum impulse was in 5th left intercostal space inside of the mid clavicular line and not diffuse. No pericardial friction sound. Border of the heart was normal. Heart sounds were strong. Rate 150/min. Cardiac rhythm was not regular. No pathological murmurs.

心　脏

心前区无鼓起，无异常脉冲或震颤。最大脉冲点位于中锁骨线内的第 5 左肋间内，未减弱。无心包摩擦音。心脏的边界正常。心音强。心率 150/ 分钟。心律不规律。无病理性杂音。

【例 3】

Chest

Chest wall: Veins could not be seen easily. No subcutaneous emphysema. Intercostal space was neither narrowed nor widened. No tenderness.

Thorax: Symmetric bilaterally. No deformities.

Breast: Symmetric bilaterally.

Lungs: Respiratory movement was bilaterally symmetric with the frequency of 23/min. Thoracic expansion and tactile fremitus were symmetric bilaterally. No pleural friction fremitus. Resonance was heard during percussion. No abnormal breath sound was heard. No wheezes. No rales.

胸

胸壁：静脉无怒张。肋间隙无增宽或变窄。无触痛。

胸廓：双侧对称。无畸形。

乳房：双侧对称。

肺：呼吸运动双侧对称，频率为 23/ 分钟，胸廓运动和触觉语颤双侧对称。无胸膜摩擦感。叩诊时可听到共鸣。无异常的呼吸声。无喘鸣。无啰音。

6.4.9 实验室数据（Laboratory Data）

1. 内容和要求

与现病史相关的实验室检查的结果均应记录在病历。实验室数据的内容一般按如下顺序排列：基础实验室检查结果、专科实验室检查结果、影像学检查结果和心电图检查结果。如果检查结果有异常，医师应进行记录并适当描述。

这部分多用一般现在时或一般过去时，有时可直接用名词词组来表示。

2. 常用表达

1）常见检查

examination of blood cell 血液细胞检查

examination of marrow cell 骨髓细胞检查

examination of hemostasis and coagulation 出血和凝血检查

kidney function examination 肾功能检查

liver function examination 肝功能检查

endocrine test 内分泌试验

immunological examination 免疫学检查

blood gas assay 血气分析

urine examination 小便检查

bacterial culture 细菌培养

ECG/EKG 心电图

MRI 核磁共振

stool examination 大便检查

fluid examination 液体检查

X-ray examination X 线检查

ultrasonography 超声波

2）常用结构

give a negative/positive result 结果阴性 / 阳性

examined item + data 检查项目 + 数据

3. 示例

【例 1】

Laboratory data: White blood cells count 5.9, hemoglobin 111 g/L, hematocrit 35.3. Sodium 142. Potassium 4.3, chloride 106, CO_2 25, BUN 2.6 mmol/L, creatinine 57 μmol/L, glucose 4.1 mmol/L. Albumin 36 g/L.

实验室数据：白细胞计数 5.9，血红蛋白 111 克 / 升，血细胞比容 35.3，钠 142，钾 4.3，氯化物 106，二氧化碳 25，尿素 2.6 毫摩尔 / 升，肌酐 57 微摩尔 / 升，葡萄糖 4.1 毫摩尔 / 升，白蛋白 36 克 / 升。

【例 2】

Laboratory data: Hemoglobin concentration is 152 g/L. Erythrocytes count is 5.1×10^{12}/L. Leukocytes count is 6.0×10^9/L. Urinalysis gives a negative test for albumin and sugar. Electrocardiogram shows right ventricular hypertrophy.

实验室数据：血红蛋白浓度为 152 克 / 升，红细胞计数 5.1×10^{12}/ 升，白细胞计数 6.0×10^9/ 升。尿常规未见尿蛋白及尿糖阴性。心电图提示右心室肥大。

【例 3】

Hb: 82 g/L. WBC: 5.5×10^9/L, with N 69%, L 28, M 3%. PIT: 3,000 × 109/L. Urinalysis is normal. X-ray barium meal shows ulcer nice and Hampton line. Gastroscopy reveals lesions near the pylorus.

血红蛋白 82 克 / 升，白细胞 5.5×10^9 / 升，N 69%，L 28，M 3%，血小板 3 000 × 10^9 / 升。尿检正常。钡餐胸片提示溃疡良好和汉姆普顿线。胃镜提示幽门区病变。

6.4.10 病史小结 / 病历摘要（History Summary）

1. 内容和要求

病史小结是指在记录完住院病历的主要内容后，将病史、体格检查、实验室检查、器械检查等主要资料简要整合并进行分析，鉴别出患者的异常症状和体征，并做出总结；重点突出阳性发现，以提示诊断的依据。

这部分一般用一般过去时或一般现在时，多用被动语态，还常用省略句。

2. 示例

【例 1】

This 83-year-old woman with a history of congestive heart failure, and coronary artery disease risk factors of hypertension and post-menopausal state presents with substernal chest pain. On exam she was found to be in sinus tachycardia, with no JVD, but there are bibasilar rales and pedal edema, suggestive of some degree of congestive heart failure. EKG changes indicate an acute anterolateral myocardial infarction, and the lab shows elevation of CPK and troponin.

这名 83 岁的女性有充血性心力衰竭病史，高血压和绝经后状态的冠心病危险因素表现为胸骨下胸痛。检查发现她窦性心动过速，无颈静脉扩张，但双肺底湿啰音和双足水肿提示一定程度的充血性心力衰竭。心电图改变提示急性前外侧心肌梗死，实验室提示肌酸激酶和肌钙蛋白升高。

【例 2】

History summary:

(1) Patient was a bank clerk, female, 45 years old.

(2) Right breast mass found for more than half a month.

(3) No special past history.

(4) Physical examination showed no abnormity in lung, heart and abdomen. Information about her breast can be seen above.

(5) Shorting of investigation information.

病史小结：

（1）患者是银行职员，女性，45 岁。

（2）右乳肿块发现半个多月。

（3）没有特殊既往史。

（4）体格检查：肺、心脏、腹部均未见异常。关于其乳房信息见前面。

（5）调查资料不足。

6.4.11 诊断 / 印象（Diagnosis/Impression）

1. 内容和要求

这部分是医生在综合分析了患者的各种情况后进行的初步诊断，在经过住院检查治疗后可做出最后诊断。初步诊断最少有一个诊断结果，但是很多时候都会有更多甚至十几个诊断结果。

这部分表述比较简单，一般用序号列出一个或多个诊断，诊断结果全部用名词短语表示。

2. 示例

【例 1】

Imp.: Acute bronchitis

印象：急性支气管炎

【例 2】

Diagnosis: Anxiety/depression/alcohol abuse

诊断：焦虑 / 抑郁 / 酗酒

【例 3】

Diagnosis:

(1) Chronic obstructive pulmonary disease exacerbation

(2) Severe aortic stenosis with congestive heart failure

(3) Severe coronary artery disease

(4) Chronic renal failure

(5) Dementia

(6) Arrhythmia

(7) Urinary tract infection with Pseudomonas

(8) Left lower lobe pneumonia

(9) Diabetes mellitus

诊断：

（1）慢性阻塞性肺病加重

（2）重度主动脉瓣狭窄伴充血性心力衰竭

（3）严重冠状动脉疾病

（4）慢性肾功能衰竭

（5）痴呆症

（6）心律失常

（7）假单胞菌尿路感染

（8）左下叶肺炎

（9）糖尿病

6.4.12 治疗（Treatment）

1. 内容和要求

治疗是病历报告中的一项重要内容，要详细记述处理意见，写明所用药物的剂型、剂量和用法；每种药物和疗法各写一行；还应注明是否需复诊及复诊要求。

这部分主要使用名词词组或省略句，语言简洁明了。

2. 示例

【例 1】

Rp:

(1) Cisapride, 15 mg t.i.d., 7d.

(2) Cimetidine, 200 mg t.i.d., 7d.

(3) Life style changes: Higher pillow (10–15 cm); no more drinking; eat less meat but more vegetables and fruits; go on physical exercise; lose weight appropriately; loosely dressed.

(4) Keep a simple mind and continue psychological consulting.

(5) Subsequent visit after 7 days.

治疗方案：

（1）西沙比利一天 3 次，每次 15 毫克，7 天。

（2）西咪替丁一天 3 次，每次 200 毫克，7 天。

（3）改变生活习惯：垫高枕头（10 ~ 15 厘米）；戒酒；少吃肉，多吃蔬菜、水果；坚持体育锻炼；适当减肥；衣着宽松舒适。

（4）不要思虑过甚，坚持心理咨询。

（5）7 天后复诊。

【例 2】

Treatment plan:

(1) Admission: Typically, oral antibiotics, rest, fluids, and home care are sufficient for complete resolution. However, the symptoms get worse, the pneumonia does not improve with home treatment, and the person will have to be hospitalized.

(2) Penicillin 400,000 u (i.m.) b.i.d. (after intradermal test): Penicillin is the usual drug of choice in the treatment of streptococcus infection.

(3) Streptomycin 0.15 (i.m.) b.i.d.: Cephalosporin is important antibiotics in the treatment of invasive infections caused by streptococcus pneumonia.

(4) Cedilanid 0.2 mg (i.m.) start. And then 0.1 mg (i.m.) every 6 hours for twice.

治疗计划：

（1）入院：通常，口服抗生素、卧床休息、多喝水、休养可以达到治愈。然而，当症状出现恶化，家庭治疗后肺炎并无缓解时，患者则需要入院治疗。

（2）青霉素 400 000 u（肌注），一天两次（皮试后）：青霉素是治疗链球菌感染的常用药。

（3）链霉素 0.15（肌注），一天两次：头孢类药物是治疗链球菌侵入性感染的重要抗生素。

（4）西地兰首剂 0.2 毫克（肌注），然后每隔 6 小时肌注两次，每次 0.1 毫克。

6.4.13 病程记录（Progress Notes）

1. 内容和要求

这部分记录患者住院期间接受的检查、治疗用药及出院时的情况，如临床治愈（cured）、好转（improved）、未改善（unchanged）、死亡（died）等。医师应及时记录并写明日期；遇到危重患者时，同一天里可能要做好几次病程记录。

这部分表述常用一般过去时和过去完成时，多用被动语态。

2. 示例

【例 1】

The patient was admitted and placed on fluid rehydration and mineral supplement. The patient improved, showing gradual resolution of nausea and vomiting. The patient was discharged in stable condition.

患者入院并接受液体补液和矿物质补充剂。患者病情好转，恶心、呕吐逐渐消退。出院时情况稳定。

【例 2】

The patient was given penicillin 400,000 u (i.m.) b.i.d. with dramatic therapeutic efficacy as her temperature (40.0 ℃) returned to normal within 24 hrs. Such symptoms as pain, cough, and rusty sputum were relieved one by one by giving penicillin, toclase, and APC. Follow-up chest film revealed the infiltration was nearly completely cleared up. WBC returned to normal limit and the patient became asymptomatic. Clinically cured, the patient was discharged.

给予青霉素 400 000 u（肌注），一天两次，具有显著疗效，患者体温（40.0 摄氏度）在 24 小时内恢复正常。疼痛、咳嗽、铁锈色痰液等症状通过给予青霉素、咳必清、阿司匹林后逐一缓解。后续胸部影片显示渗透几乎完全被清除。白细胞计数恢复正常，患者无症状。临床治愈后，患者出院。

6.4.14 出院小结（Discharge Summary）

1. 内容和要求

患者出院时由医师书写出院小结，以便复诊和随访时参考。住院小结应参考出院记录书写，说明患者入院前后的病情、检查、诊断、治疗的要点，以及出院时的情况、出院时间、住院日期、出院诊断、出院医嘱要点等。

2. 示例

Name: XXX

Age: 73 years old

Sex: Male

Admission Date: XXX

Operation Date: XXX

Discharge Date: XXX

Diagnosis:

Acute myocardial infraction

Type 2 diabetes mellitus

Admission: Sudden chest pain for 4 hours

Patient History: 73-year-old man without significant heart problems presented with sudden chest pain for 4 hours. And the pain constantly radiated to the shoulder and back. The ECG of the patient showed the ST segment of the leads Ⅱ, Ⅲ, AVF raised 0.1–0.2 mv and was admitted for further evaluation and treatment.

Physical Examination: Blood pressure 120/60 mmHg, Pulse 60/minute. The lungs were clear. The heart rate was regular, 60 beats per minute. No murmur and pericardial rub were heard. There was no peripheral edema.

Laboratory Results:

Hb: 133 g/L　　　　Glucose: 8.6 mmol/L (< 6.1)

CHOL: 4.68 mmol/L　　TG: 0.86 mmol/L

LDL-C: 3.07 mmol/L　　HDL: 1.11 mmol/L

CRP: 8.60 mg/L (0–8 mg/L)　　CK-MB: 299.2 U/L (0–16 U/L)

Troponin I: 0.24 ng/mL (< 0.04 ng/mL)

ECG: A normal rhythm at rate of 60/minute, ST segment raised 0.1–0.2 mv in leads Ⅱ, Ⅲ, AVF.

Transthoracic Echocardiogram (TTE): The size of left atrium is 41.2 mm and the other chambers were normal. EF: 51%

CAG: The middle of right coronary artery (RCA) completely blocked and left coronary artery (LCA) has a 50% lesion in the proximal and left anterior descending (LAD) has some 30%–50% lesions. After admission, we implant one stent (3.5/15 mm) in the RCA.

Treatment: After operation, treatment was started for the recovery. It was treated with Aspirin 100 mg po q.d., Plavix 75 mg po q.d., Dilatrend 6.25 mg bid, Imdur 60 mg q.d., and Clexane (low-molecular-weight heparins sodium) 5,000 Usc q12h. After 16 days of recovery, the patient is well. So we think the patient can be discharged from hospital.

Medication:

(1) Medicines to improve heart function

Aspirin 100 mg

Plavix 75 mg for 9 months

Zocor (statin) 40 mg

Micardis 40 mg

Spironolactone 20 mg

Dilatrend 6.25 mg

(2) Medicines to control blood sugar

Glargine (insulin) 34 U ih

Glucobay 50 mg

Avandia 8 mg

Comments:

(1) No smoking and drinking, and keep diet.

(2) Strictly control blood sugar.

(3) Be attentive to keeping rest and do not do high-intensity exercises.

(4) Take medicines on time and follow-up visit after one month.

姓名：XXX

年龄：73 岁

性别：男

入院日期：XXX

手术日期：XXX

出院日期：XXX

诊断：

急性心肌梗死

Ⅱ型糖尿病

入院：猝发性胸痛 4 小时

患者病史：73 岁男性，无明显心脏问题，出现突发性胸痛 4 小时。疼痛不断放射到肩膀和背部。患者心电图显示 ST 段在导联 II、III、AVF 中升高 0.1 ~ 0.2 毫伏，入院进一步评估和治疗。

体格检查：血压 120/60 毫米汞柱，脉搏 60/分钟。肺部清楚。心率有规律，每分钟 60 次。未听到杂音和心包摩擦音。无外周水肿。

检查结果：

血红蛋白：133 克 / 升

葡萄糖：8.6 毫摩尔 / 升（< 6.1）

胆固醇：4.68 毫摩尔 / 升

甘油三酯：0.86 毫摩尔 / 升

低密脂蛋白：3.07 毫摩尔 / 升

高密度脂蛋白：1.11 毫摩尔 / 升

C 反应性蛋白：8.60 毫克 / 升（0 ~ 8 毫克 / 升）

肌酸激酶：299.2 U/L（0 ~ 16 U/L）

肌钙蛋白 I：0.24 纳克 / 毫升（< 0.04 纳克 / 毫升）

心电图：心律正常，速率为 60/分钟，ST 段在导联 II、III、AVF 中升高 0.1 ~ 0.2 毫伏。

经胸超声心动图：左心房大小为 41.2 毫米，其他腔室正常。EF：51%

冠状动脉造影：右冠状动脉的中间完全闭塞，左冠状动脉在近端有 50% 的病变，左前降有大约 30% ~ 50% 的病变。入院后在右冠状动脉中植入一个支架（3.5/15 毫米）。

治疗：手术后，开始治疗使其恢复。用阿司匹林每日 100 毫克，口服；波立维每日 75 毫克，口服；达利全 6.25 毫克，每日两次；依姆多每日 60 毫克，口服和克赛（低分子量肝素钠）5 000 皮下注射单位，每 12 小时一次。经过 16 天的康复，患者身体健康。因此我们认为，患者可以出院。

药物：

（1）改善心脏功能的药物

阿司匹林 100 毫克，口服

波立维 75 毫克，口服，持续 9 个月

辛伐他汀（他汀类药物）40 毫克，口服

美卡素 40 毫克，口服

螺内酯 20 毫克，口服

达利全 6.25 毫克，口服

（2）控制血糖的药物

甘精胰岛素 34 U ih

拜糖平 50 毫克，口服

文迪雅 8 毫克，口服

指导：

（1）禁止吸烟和饮酒，并保持饮食。

（2）严格控制血糖。

（3）注意保持休息，不要做高强度的运动。

（4）按时吃药，1 个月后随访。

Exercises

Exercise I　Translate the following into English.

1. 饭后两小时感到上腹痛，痛感时隐时现，持续两年。
2. 患者休息时感觉心绞痛，睡眠期间有精神压力，症状持续一周以上。
3. 咳嗽之后几分钟出现剧烈头痛，血压升高。
4. 患者否认有哮喘和肺炎，过去也未发现对青霉素过敏。
5. 主诉：最近三天出现黑色柏油便，上腹痛加剧。

Exercise II　Translate the following into Chinese.

1. The stools have been kind of sandy color, not loose. Urine has been sort of like tea. His abdomen has been kind of swollen. Eyes were yellowish. Some thick, rusty colored sputum was brought up when he coughed.

2. P.I.: Male, age 64, had been a diabetic for the past four years, controlled on diet. He was well until three months ago when he became somewhat weaker than previously. His status remained the same until two weeks ago when he had minor eyelid operation and doctors at that time noticed an elevated bold sugar. He was noted to have a ++++ sugar in the urine with a negative acetone. This morning he was noted to be agitated and confused and uncommunicative.

3. Her bowel movement is irregular. Water is normal. Period finished two years ago. No chills. She feels weak, and has put on 4 pounds of weight in the last three months. She has had burning pain for two years. Thick taste of sour liquid in mouth. Blenching a little, no vomiting.

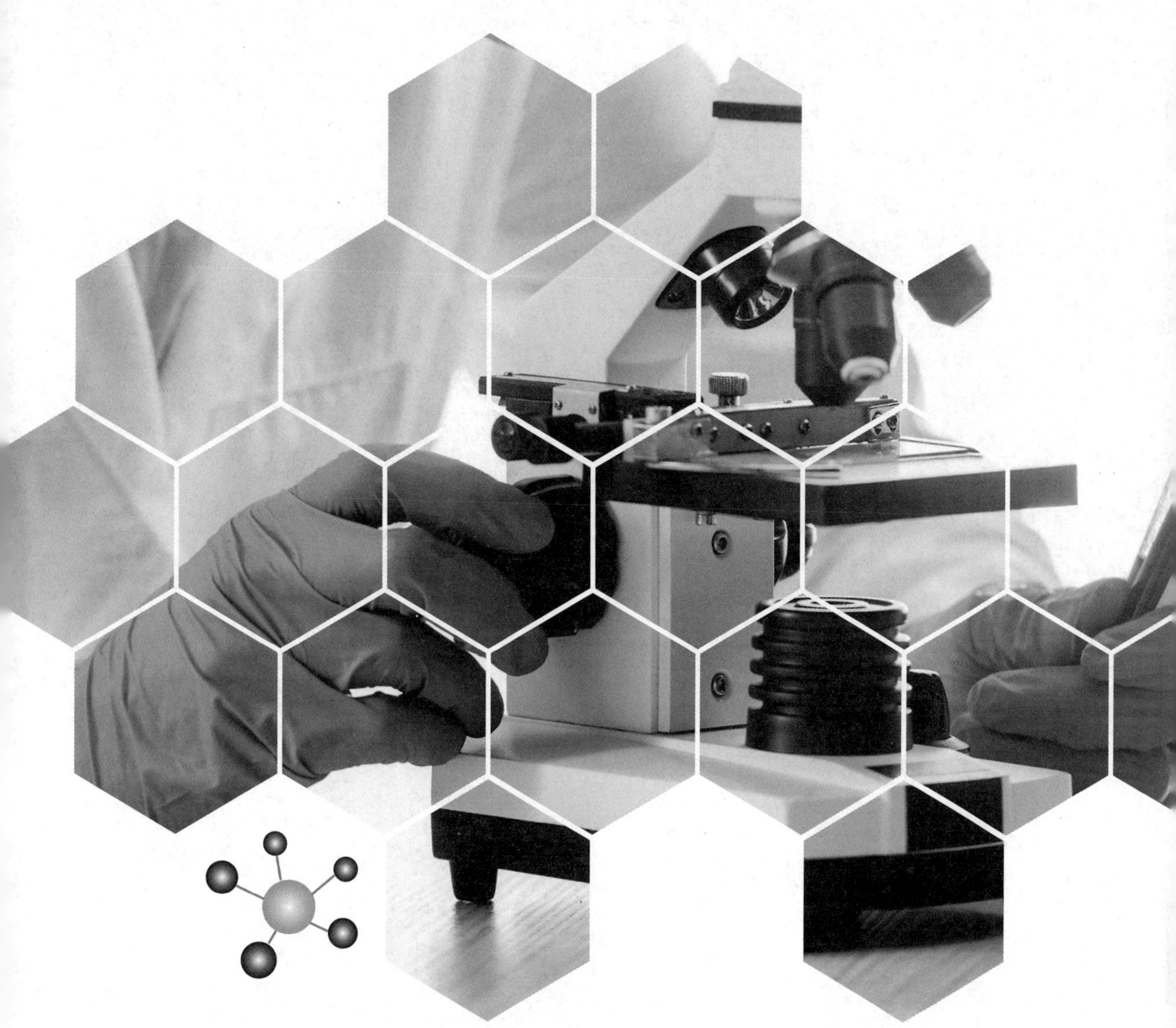

学术篇

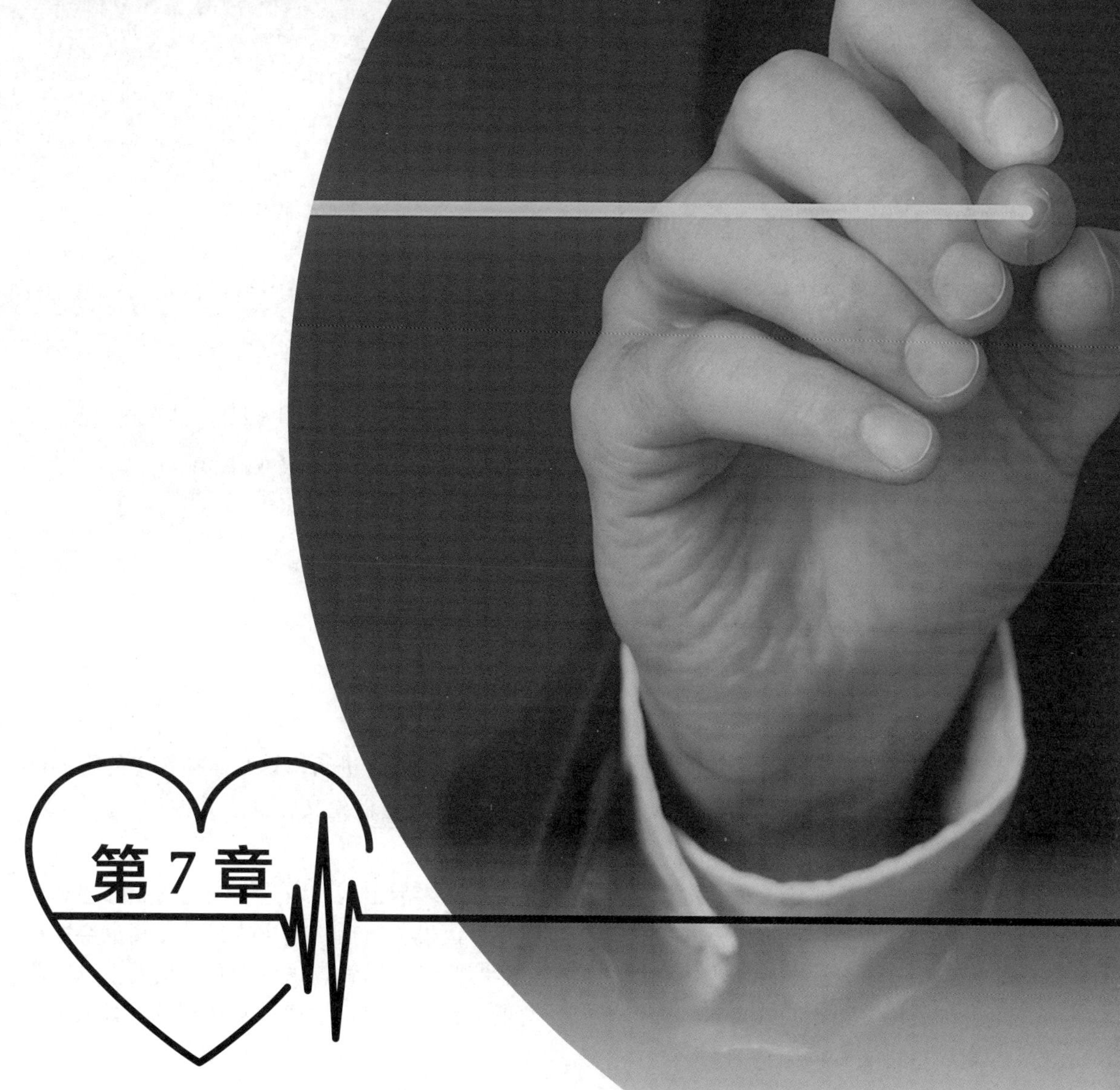

第 7 章

医学论文标题与摘要（Titles and Abstracts of Medical Papers）

Prevention is better than cure.

预防胜于治疗。

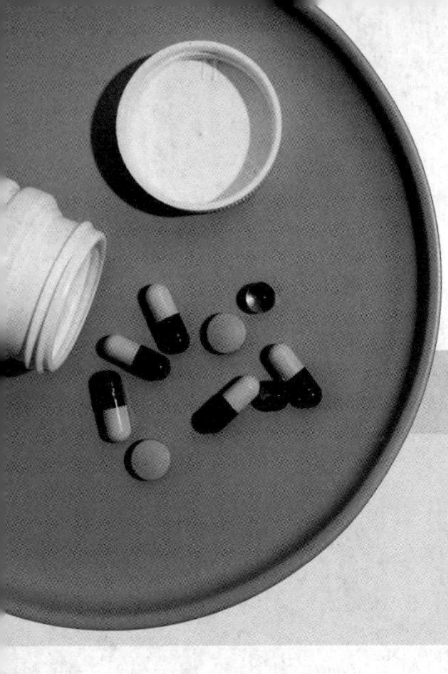

Warm-up

1. How many kinds of abstracts can you choose to use?
2. Please list the basic requirements of writing a title.

标题是一篇论文的点睛之笔，亦可被称为题目、篇名、文题等，以语言准确简洁为特点，用特定内容和简明形式对论文要义及中心思想进行提炼与概括。它的重要性在于它通常是一篇论文留给读者的第一印象，也是这篇论文区别于其他论文的标志，影响着一篇论文被检索的程度。

摘要是一篇论文内容的浓缩与精华，在正文之前出现，对论文进行简要陈述和概括，为读者提供论文的基本梗概，具有独立、代表、概括和报告的特点。其重要性在于它呈现了论文的基本内容和研究框架，能够为信息检索提供免费且有用的信息。联合国教科文组织明确规定“全世界公开发表的论文，无论用何种文字写成，必须附一篇简短的英文摘要”。

7.1 标题与摘要写作的基本要求（Basic Requirements of Writing Titles and Abstracts）

7.1.1 标题撰写的基本要求（Basic Requirements of Writing Titles）

撰写标题是一门重要的艺术和技术，标题的撰写应尽量达到以下要求：

（1）准确（accuracy）：标题能精准反应论文的内容、研究范围、深度、独创性和特色、用词准确；标题中所使用的数字、公式、符号、方程式等都应符合文献标引及目录检索要求，避免个人独创的非公认的缩略语或公式符号等情况的出现。

（2）简洁（brevity）：标题能用最少的文字概括最主要的内容、呈现最大的信息量；一般为 10 ~ 12 个单词或者不超过 100 个英文字符。

（3）醒目（catchy）：标题应居于文章的醒目位置，尽量将表达文章核心内容的中心词放在最突出的位置。

（4）概括（recapitulative）：标题应全面、完整的反映文章内容。

（5）便于检索（easy to retrieve）：标题应准确、简洁、概括、便于检索。

7.1.2 摘要撰写的基本要求（Basic Requirements of Writing Abstracts）

摘要是论文的高度凝练，具体应参考以下要求：

（1）字数适当：《美国医学协会杂志》规定摘要不超过 350 词，我国编辑标准要求摘要为 200 ~ 300 词。总体来说，摘要字数不宜过多，200 字左右即可。

（2）格式正确：摘要的分类有多种，其格式都有一定的要求。无论采用哪类摘要，作者均应保证其格式的正确性。

（3）逻辑清晰：摘要应注意逻辑清晰，使读者快速、准确地获取论文的研究思路、方法、材料、数据、研究结果和研究要义。

（4）语言精练：摘要措辞应精练清晰，直观表达研究过程、方法、结论等。

7.2 标题与摘要的分类、格式与书写（Classification, Formatting, and Writing of Titles and Abstracts）

7.2.1 标题的分类（Classification of Titles）

医学论文的标题可以只有正标题，也可以正副标题均出现。正标题是最普通、最常见的形式，应符合准确、简洁、醒目、概括、便于检索的特点。副标题是对正标题的补充说明，通常放在正标题之后或之下，突出和强调论文某一重要方面的内容，如研究方法、重点、范围等。具体使用何种格式，作者需要考虑论文内容及发表杂志要求。

7.2.2 标题的格式（Formatting of Titles）

正标题的格式有多种类型，每种类型的具体书写格式又有不同。正标题突出的是文章重点，常包含最核心的关键词。

副标题的格式可以和正标题相同或不同，正副标题常以冒号或者破折号分开。副标题的使用在国外期刊中较多见。

1. 正标题的格式

正标题的格式通常含短语型和句子型。医学论文的英语标题以短语构成较多，少数采用句子，而在句子型标题中，陈述句居多，也可用疑问句。

1）短语型标题格式

（1）名词短语型标题

名词短语型标题由一个或多个名词或复合名词加上前位或后位的必要修饰成分构成，通常没有逗号或句号，多有以下几种形式：

- **名词 + 介词**

  Postoperative Syndromes **After** Liver Surgery

  肝脏术后综合征

- **名词 + 分词（过去分词 -ed、现在分词 -ing）**

  Thyroid Carcinoma **Induced** by Irradiation for Hodgkin's Disease

  霍奇金病放射治疗引起的甲状腺癌

- **名词 + 不定式**

  Suggestion **to Abolish** Icterus Index Determination Where Quantitative Bilirubin Assay Is Available

  建议在可进行胆红素定量检测的情况下取消黄疸指数测定

- **名词 + 同位语**

  Social Network Analysis of Tourism Data: **A Case Study** of Quarantine Decisions in COVID-19 Pandemic

  旅游数据的社会网络分析：新冠肺炎大流行中检疫决策的案例研究

- **名词 + 从句**

  Factors **that** Predict Outcome of Abdominal Operations in Patients with Advanced Cirrhosis

  晚期肝硬化患者腹部手术后的预测因素

- **定语 + 名词**

  COVID-19 **Research** in LMICs

  中低收入国家新冠肺炎研究

（2）-ing 分词短语型标题

Strengthening the Global Effort on COVID-19 Research

加强全球新冠肺炎研究工作

（3）介词短语型标题

On the Pearls and Perils of Subspecialization

论亚专业化的利弊

（4）动词不定式短语作中心词型标题

To Protect Those Who Serve

保护服务人员

2）句子型标题格式

句子型标题具有完整的主谓结构，标题的中心词即句子的主语，而谓语则采用简单形式。句子型标题分为简单句型标题和复合句型标题，这两种标题又可以继续细分。

（1）简单句型标题

简单句型标题指标题句中只有一个主谓（系）结构或动宾结构，可以是陈述句或疑问句。

- 陈述句

陈述句型标题描述某事或陈述某人对某事或某个问题的看法或观点，可分为肯定句和否定句。我们应注意这类标题末尾不加标点。

a. 肯定句

Tribbles Pseudokinase 3 **Inhibits** the Adipogenic Differentiation of Human Adipose-Derived Mesenchymals Tribbles

同源蛋白 3 抑制人脂肪间充质干细胞成脂分化

b. 否定句

Attenuated Early Pregnancy Weight Gain by Prenatal Lifestyle Interventions **Does Not** Prevent Gestational Diabetes in the LIFE-Moms Consortium

在生命母亲联盟中，通过产前生活方式干预减轻妊娠早期体重增加并不能预防妊娠糖尿病

- 疑问句

能够作标题的英文疑问句型只有一般疑问句和特殊疑问句，可以是完整结构或者是省略结构，句末一般用问号。

a. 一般疑问句

Is a Change of Factor VIII Product a Risk Factor for the Development of a Factor VIII Inhibitor?

凝血因子 VIII 产物的变化是产生凝血因子 VIII 抑制剂的危险因素吗?

b. 特殊疑问句

How Well Are Dental Qualitative Studies Involving Interviews and Focus Groups Reported?

涉及访谈和焦点小组的牙科定性研究报告的效果如何?

c. 完整型疑问句标题

Is Sclerotherapy Better than Intralesional Excision for Treating Aneurysmal Bone Cysts?

硬化疗法治疗动脉瘤样骨囊肿优于病灶切除吗?

d. 省略型疑问句标题

Vitamin E: Too Much or Not Enough?

维生素 E：太多了还是不足?

注意：有一种特殊情况，即疑问代词或疑问副词 + 不定式结构，这种结构起到的是名词作用，因此这种结构作标题不加问号，如 What to Pay Attention to When You Got COVID-19。

（2）复合句型标题

复合句型标题是指在标题中有两个或两个以上从属关系的主谓结构的句子型标题，如带有定语从句的复合句型标题 [这种标题中包含：主谓结构 + 定语从句（主谓结构）]；又如带有宾语从句或状语从句的复合句型标题。

- 带有定语从句的标题

  Turnover of Thrombomodulin at the Cell Surface **Occurs** at a Similar Rate to Receptors **that Are** Not Actively Internalized

  细胞表面凝血调节蛋白以与受体相同的速度更新并非由于自动进行的内转换作用所致

- 带有宾语从句的标题

  Are Physicians Aware **Which** of Their Patients Have Indwelling Urinary Catheters?

  医生们知道哪个患者留置导尿管吗?

- 带有状语从句的标题

  If You Should Live Long, Choose Your Parents Well

  要想活得长，选好父母

2. 副标题的格式

副标题的格式与主标题可以相同，也可以不同。正副标题之间常以冒号或圆点隔开，也可以各自独立。当正标题只有第一个单词的首字母大写时，副标题中的首个单词的首字母可大写，也可小写。副标题的主要作用是补充说明，说明内容主要分为以下几种：

1）突出病例数：强调研究样本以增强说服力或强调罕见性

Free composite groin flap to solve a complex loss of tissue in a traumatic injury of the foot: **A case report**

游离复合腹股沟皮瓣解决创伤性足部复杂的组织损失：一个病例报告

Solitary fibrous tumor of thyroid: **A case report with review of literature**

甲状腺孤立性纤维性肿瘤：一篇带有文献回顾的病例报告

2）突出重点内容：强调同类事物中的核心部分

Functional gastrointestinal disorders: **History, pathophysiology, and clinical features**

功能性胃肠疾病：病史、病理生理学和临床特征

3）突出研究方法：强调某种方法的优劣或重要性

Diabetes after infectious hepatitis: **A follow-up study**

传染性肝炎继发糖尿病患者随访调查

4）提出疑问：启发读者，用争论和质疑吸引读者参与共同探讨

Immunosuppression in Autoimmune Hepatitis: **Is There an End Game?**

自身免疫性肝炎的免疫抑制：研究何时方休？

5）说明研究时间：反映出某一特定疾病的短期波动、变化规律、周期性趋势，是某些特定医学研究的重要一面

Bronchiolitis Epidemics in France During the SARS-CoV-2 Pandemic: **The 2020–2021 and 2021–2022 Seasons**

严重急性呼吸系统综合征冠状病毒 2 型大流行期间法国毛细支气管炎的流行：2020—2021 年和 2021—2022 年

6）用同位语：表示强调

Alzheimer's Disease: **An Emerging Affliction of Aging Population**

阿尔茨默病是老年人群中新兴的疾病

7）表示长篇连载论文的分篇主题

Medical Treatment of Early Breast Cancer I: **Adjuvant Treatment**

Medical Treatment of Early Breast Cancer II: **Endocrine Therapy**

Medical Treatment of Early Breast Cancer III: **Chemotherapy**

早期乳腺癌的药物治疗 I：辅助治疗

早期乳腺癌的药物治疗 II：内分泌治疗

早期乳腺癌的药物治疗 III：化疗

7.2.3 标题的书写（Writing of Titles）

尽管标题分类多种多样，但作者在拟定标题时应明白标题结构并非越复杂越好，而是应遵循准确、简洁、概括、醒目、便于检索的基本要求。常见的标题书写方式如下：

1）大写所有字母

HOW TO PREVENET RENEL TRAUMA

2）大写首个单词的首字母

Machine learning-based scoring system to predict in-hospital outcomes in patients hospitalized with COVID-19

3）大写所有实词的首字母

Lifestyle Changes and Psychological Well-Being in Older Adults During COVID-19 Pandemic

7.2.4 摘要的分类（Classification of Abstracts）

基于不同的研究内容和研究方法，论文摘要的结构会有所不同。

按格式分类，摘要可分为结构式摘要（structured abstract）和非结构式摘要（non-structured abstract）。

按性质分类，摘要可分为报道性摘要（informative abstract）、指示性摘要（indicative abstract）、报道－指示性摘要（informative-indicative abstract）、结构式摘要（structured abstract）。下面主要对四种摘要的格式进行讲解。

7.2.5 摘要的格式（Formatting of Abstracts）

1. 报道性摘要的格式

报道性摘要又称资料性摘要、信息性摘要，从结构和内容上来说，报道性摘要包含如下信息：

（1）研究背景（context/background）;

（2）研究目的（objective/purpose）;

（3）研究方法（methods）;

（4）研究过程与结果（发现）（procedure and result of the research）;

（5）结论和建议（conclusion and suggestions）;

（6）对未来的展望（future prospects）。

报道性摘要不是简单的原文缩减，其语言精练、简明准确、信息量大、参考价值高，阅读摘要可以部分取代阅读原文。学术性期刊或论文集多选用此种摘要，词数一般为300左右。

根据陈述内容的不同，报道性摘要在时态运用上也有所不同。介绍背景时用一般现在时、现在完成时；说明研究目的时用一般现在时、现在完成时或一般过去时；讲述研究过程和结果时用一般过去时；结论和建议部分用一般现在时；展望部分用一般现在时或一般将来时。

【例】

青年男性心脏病发作（心肌梗死）经验的定性研究

摘要

目标： 心脏病发作或心肌梗死（MI）在社会心理学领域的影响在年轻人中可能特别严重，对他们来说，严重的健康事件是不正常的。在西方国家，心肌梗死发病率正在下降，但在英格兰，45 岁以下人群的心肌梗死人数已趋于平稳，其中约 90% 的患者是男性。关于年轻人心肌梗死经历的定性研究有限，没有一项研究专门针对 45 岁以下的人进行抽样。这项研究的目的是了解 45 岁以下的男性人群是如何适应和理解 MI 的。**设计：** 基于半结构化深入访谈的定性研究设计。**方法：** 有目的地招募和采访了 10 名在过去 3 ~ 6 个月内经历过心肌梗死的 45 岁以下男性。访谈被逐字记录下来，并使用解释性现象学分析进行分析。**结果：** 确定了七个高级主题。这篇文章深入探讨了三个最具原创性的主题：①“我不是一个男人”，它描述了 MI 后失去“男性”（力量、独立性、提供能力）的经历；②“缩短的视野”，涵盖参与者对未来的预见和随后重新排序的感觉；③“生活失去了色彩”，描述了生活方式变化带来的愉悦感的丧失。**结论：** 主题与关于年轻人心肌梗死的定性文献大致重叠。然而，一些主题（如心肌梗死后“男性”的丧失，以及对心肌梗死风险因素的矛盾心理）似乎是本研究独有的。讨论主题还涉及焦虑和抑郁的危险因素，以及这可能如何为年轻男性人群的临床护理提供信息。关于这个主题已经知道了什么？英格兰 45 岁以下人群的心肌梗死发病率并未下降。适应 MI 对年轻人来说尤其具有挑战性，这也许是因为它不规范。然而，对于年轻人患心肌梗死的经历知之甚少。这项研究增加了什么？这是首次对 45 岁以下的 MI 患者进行定性研究，从而绘制出流行病学趋势图，进一步支持现有青年 MI 文献中确定的一些主题。这里确定了新的主题，可以为该人群的临床护理提供相关见解。

关键词： 调整；心脏病发作；解释现象学分析；心肌梗死；质量的；幼小的

A Qualitative Study of Younger Men's Experience of Heart Attack (Myocardial Infarction)

Abstract

Objectives: The effects of heart attack, or myocardial infarction (MI), across psychosocial domains may be particularly acute in younger adults, for whom serious health events are non-normative. MI morbidity is declining in Western countries, but in England MI numbers have plateaued for the under-45 cohort, where approximately 90% of patients are male. Qualitative research on younger adults' experience of MI is limited, and no study has sampled exclusively under-45s. This study aimed to understand how a sample of men under 45 adjusted to and made sense of MI. **Design:** Qualitative research design based on semi-structured in-depth interviews. **Methods:** Ten men aged under 45 who had experienced MI in the past 3–6 months were purposively recruited and interviewed. Interviews were transcribed verbatim and analyzed using interpretative phenomenological analysis. **Results:** Seven superordinate themes were identified. This article focuses in depth on the three most original themes: ① "I'm less of a man", which described experiences of losing "maleness" (strength, independence, ability to provide) post-MI; ② "Shortened horizons", which covered participants' sense of foreshortened future and consequent reprioritization; and ③ "Life loses its color", describing the loss of pleasure from lifestyle-related changes. **Conclusion:** Themes broadly overlapped with the qualitative literature on younger adult MI. However, some themes (e.g., loss of "maleness" post-MI, and ambivalence towards MI risk factors) appeared unique to this study. Themes were also discussed in relation to risk factors for anxiety and depression, and how this might inform clinical care for a younger, male population. What is already known on this subject? Myocardial infarction morbidity is not declining in England for under-45s. Adjustment to MI is particularly challenging for younger adults, perhaps because it is non-normative. However, little is known about the experience of MI in younger adults. What does this study add? This is the first qualitative study to sample MI patients exclusively under 45, thereby mapping to epidemiological trends. Further support is provided for some themes identified in the existing young adult MI literature. New themes are identified here which can provide insights relevant to clinical care in this population.

Keywords: adjustment; heart attack; interpretative phenomenological analysis; myocardial infarction; qualitative; young

这篇摘要的第一部分主要介绍本文的研究背景和目标，用一般现在时表达，个别地方使用一般过去时；第二、第三、第四部分讲研究设计、方法和结果，用一般过去时表达；第五部分讲结论，用一般过去时、一般现在时表达。

2. 指示性摘要的格式

指示性摘要也称描述性摘要（descriptive abstract）或说明性摘要、论点摘要（topic abstract）。指示性摘要一般只提示论文的主题，言简意赅，信息量少，一般只用 1 ~ 2 个句子、100 个词左右，不介绍研究方法、材料、数据、结果等内容。

许多专业杂志在其目录页的标题下都有一个指示性摘要，特别是在作者认为比较重要的文章标题后。

【例】

论原发性胃肠道淋巴瘤

本文综述了治疗原发于胃肠道淋巴瘤的主要经验，并就该病的临床、病理及治疗等问题进行了讨论。

Primary Lymphomas of the Gastrointestinal Tract

An institutional experience with primary gastrointestinal lymphoma (PGL) is reviewed. The clinical, pathologic, and therapeutic aspects of PGL are discussed.

3. 报道－指示性摘要

报道－指示性摘要是一种综合性摘要，兼顾两种摘要的写法，对比较重要的、信息价值较高的内容采用报道性的形式表述，对不重要的部分以指示性的形式概括一下；词数为 200 左右。

【例】

2019 年新型冠状病毒肺炎的 CT 影像学研究进展

摘要：高传染性的新型冠状病毒病（COVID-19）于 2019 年年底爆发，至今已持续近 1 年，该大流行在世界各地仍然猖獗。COVID-19 的诊断是在流行病学史、临床症状、实验室和影像学检查的基础上进行的。其中，影像学检查对临床疑似病例患者的诊断、无症状感染的调查及家系聚类、患者恢复情况的判断、疾病复发后的再诊断、预后预测等具有重要意义。本文就 COVID-19 大流行中 CT 影像学检查的研究进展进行了综述。

关键词：胸片；计算机断层成像；诊断；新型冠状病毒；肺炎

Progress of CT Imaging Research on
Novel Coronavirus Pneumonia in 2019

Abstract: The highly contagious novel coronavirus disease 2019 (COVID-19) broke out at the end of 2019 and has lasted for nearly one year, and the pandemic is still rampant around the world. The diagnosis of COVID-19 is on the basis of the combination of epidemiological history, clinical symptoms, and laboratory and imaging examinations. Among them, imaging examination is of importance in the diagnosis of patients with suspected clinical cases, the investigation of asymptomatic infections and family clustering, the judgment of patient recovery, rediagnosis after disease recurrence, and prognosis prediction. This article reviews the research progress of CT imaging examination in the COVID-19 pandemic.

Keywords: chest radiograph; computed tomography; diagnosis; novel coronavirus; pneumonia

4. 结构式摘要的格式

1987 年 4 月,《内科学年鉴》(*Annals of Internal Medicine*)杂志率先刊出结构式摘要的使用建议，并于同期开始使用。由于结构式摘要具有内容完整、重点突出、信息量大等特点，迄今一直被多种医学期刊或编辑采纳。不同期刊的结构式摘要在项目上存在差异，根据要求可以采用全结构式摘要（full-structured abstract）或半结构式摘要（semi-structured abstract）。

全结构式摘要由海恩斯（Haynes）博士提出，一般包含八个要素：目的（aim/objective/purpose）、设计（design）、环境（setting）、对象（patients/participants/subjects）、处置方法（interventions）、主要测定项目（main outcome measures）、结果（results）、结论（conclusion）。

【例 1】

Stress-Related Disorders of Family Members of Patients Admitted to the Intensive Care Unit with COVID-19

Abstract

Importance: The psychological symptoms associated with having a family member admitted to the intensive care unit (ICU) during the COVID-19 pandemic are not well defined.

Objective: To examine the prevalence of symptoms of stress-related disorders, primarily posttraumatic stress disorder (PTSD), in family members of patients admitted to the ICU with COVID-19 approximately 90 days after admission.

Design, Setting, and Participants: This prospective, multisite, mixed-methods observational cohort study assessed 330 family members of patients admitted to the ICU (except in New York City, which had a random sample of 25% of all admitted patients per month) between February 1 and July 31, 2020, at 8 academic-affiliated and 4 community-based hospitals in 5 U.S. states.

Exposure: Having a family member in the ICU with COVID-19.

Main Outcomes and Measures: Symptoms of PTSD at 3 months, as defined by a score of 10 or higher on the Impact of Events Scale 6 (IES-6).

Results: A total of 330 participants [mean (SD) age, 51.2 (15.1) years; 228 (69.1%) women; 150 (52.8%) White; 92 (29.8%) Hispanic] were surveyed at the 3-month time point. Most individuals were the patients' child [129 (40.6%)] or spouse or partner [81 (25.5%)]. The mean (SD) IES-6 score at 3 months was 11.9 (6.1), with 201 of 316 respondents (63.6%) having scores of 10 or higher, indicating significant symptoms of PTSD. Female participants had an adjusted mean IES-6 score of 2.6 points higher (95% CI, 1.4–3.8; $P<0.001$) than male participants, whereas Hispanic participants scored a mean of 2.7 points higher compared with non-Hispanic participants (95% CI, 1.0–4.3; $P = 0.002$). Those with graduate school experience had an adjusted mean score of 3.3 points lower (95% CI, 1.5–5.1; $P<0.001$) compared with those with up to a high school degree or equivalent. Qualitative analyses found no substantive differences in the emotional or communication-related experiences between those with high vs low PTSD scores, but those with higher scores exhibited more distrust of practitioners.

Conclusions and Relevance: In this cohort study, symptoms of PTSD among family members of ICU patients with COVID-19 were high. Hispanic ethnicity and female are associated with higher symptoms. Those with higher scores reported more distrust of practitioners.

注意:《内科学年鉴》现行的结构式摘要标题词变更为 Importance; Objective; Design, Setting, and Participants; Interventions; Main Outcomes and Measures; Results; Conclusions and Relevance。

半结构式摘要包括目的（Objective）、方法（Methods）、结果（Results）和结论（Conclusions）。

目的：说明论文要解决的问题。"目的"一般用 Objective/Purpose/Aim 来表达，常用单数形式。单数表示目的主要用动词不定式短语。

方法：说明研究设计、研究性质、研究对象及选择标准、随机分组方法、处理方法、观察手段、统计分析等。"方法"一般用 Methods 来表达，常用复数形式。句中动词用一般过去时或过去完成时，多用被动语态。

结果：主要表述研究所获得的客观或与研究结论有关的重要结果。如有可能，作者应提供具体数据和统计学资料。"结果"一般用 Results 来表达，常用复数。由于研究实验结果是回顾性陈述，因此句中动词常用一般过去时，多用被动语态。

结论：说明主要结论，包括理论意义、直接的或可能的临床应用意义。"结论"一般用 Conclusion(s) 来表达。如果结论具有普遍性，用一般现在时；如果是研究结束时的结论，不具备普遍性，则用一般过去时。

【例 2】

Factor V Leiden and PTG20210A Gene Mutation in Patients with Venous Thrombosis and Healthy Blood Donors

Abstract

Objective: To evaluate the incidence of factor V Leiden and prothrombin gene

G20210A mutation in patients with venous thrombosis and healthy volunteers.

Methods: Factor V Leiden and prothrombin gene G20210A mutation were analyzed in 97 cases of venous thrombosis and 100 healthy volunteers with the methods of one-step PCR-RFLP.

Results: PCR products for the factor V gene (175 bp) and for the prothrombin gene (118 bp) were identified to 157 bp and 98 bp fragments by electrophoreses after Taq I treatment. No factor V Leiden and prothrombin gene G20210A mutation were found in either group.

Conclusion: The low incidence of factor V Leiden and prothrombin gene G20210A mutation suggests that they are not the major genetic risk factors for thrombophilia in the Chinese.

这篇半结构式摘要包含目的、方法、结果、结论四个层次，研究目的用不定式短语表达，研究方法和结果用一般过去时表达，结论用一般现在时表达。

无论是全结构式摘要还是半结构式摘要，都包含四个“W”和一个“H”等要素：① Why did you start?（交代为什么要研究）；② What did you do?（交代研究什么）；③ How did you get results?（交代如何研究）；④ What did you find?（交代研究发现）；⑤ What does it mean?（指出研究结果及意义）。

7.2.6 摘要的书写（Writing of Abstracts）

1. 摘要的书写句型

由前文可见，医学论文摘要的分类有多种，但其包含的主要内容（如目的、方法、结果、结论等）的表达均有一些常用的书写句型。

1）表达目的（Objective/Aim）

目的部分应简洁明了、完整科学、方便检索。根据期刊的具体要求，目的部分可以用完整句描述，也可以用不定式描述。

（1）完整句类常用结构

The purpose (objective) is/ was to...

目的在于……

The primary purpose of the study is/was to...

本研究的主要目的是……

【例 1】

The purpose of this study was to examine the association between the COVID-19 vaccine and the symptoms of high fever after catching COVID-19.

本研究的目的是探讨新冠疫苗与感染新冠后高烧症状之间的关联。

The study was designed/intended to...

本研究的目的是……

The study is an attempt to...

本研究试图……

【例 2】

The study was designed/intended to research the problems about venous transfusion in out-patient clinic so as to improve the quality of nursing.

本研究旨在探讨门诊静脉输液中的问题，以提高护理质量。

主语 + 谓语 + for the purpose of...

【例 3】

The study is for the purpose of improving the effect of COVID-19 vaccine.

本研究目的是提高新冠疫苗的接种效果。

注意： study 的用法比较特殊，当它与表示研究方法的前置定语连用时，一般用单数，如 non-experimental study（非实验研究）、comparative study（比较研究）、retrospective study（回顾性研究）。当它与表示研究对象的前置定语连用时，往往用复数，如 lymphocyte studies（淋巴细胞的研究）、hemodynamic studies（血流动力学的研究）。

（2）不定式类常用结构

to + 动词，意思是"为了……"，如 to study/explore/examine/investigate（研究 / 探讨）。

【例 1】

To study the effect of overdose vs. underdose on ventricular tachyarrhythmia or death.

研究过量用药与用药不足对室性快速型心律失常或死亡的影响。

to evaluate/judge/validate/appraise/estimate/calculate/appreciate 评估 / 评价 / 验证 / 计算

to illustrate/explain/elucidate / find out 说明 / 解释 / 阐明 / 发现

【例 2】

To evaluate the efficacy and safety of high-dose penicillin as a treatment option in patients with heart disease.

评估高剂量青霉素作为心脏病患者治疗选择的有效性和安全性。

to report/present/describe 介绍 / 报道

【例 3】

To report the result of observation of the rabies vaccine influence on the recovery of pneumonia patients.

报道狂犬病疫苗对肺炎患者康复影响的观察结果。

to seek/find/ look for / search for / find out 寻找

【例 4】

To seek the combined association of diet and physical activity with AD risk.

探讨饮食与运动相结合对阿尔茨海默病患病风险的影响。

to compare/correlate/associate/ contrast... with 比较 / 对比

【例 5】

To compare the clinical efficacy and adverse reaction between Everolimus and Axitinib as the second-line treatment of metastatic renal cell carcinoma (mRCC).

比较依维莫司与阿昔替尼二线治疗转移性肾细胞癌的临床疗效及不良反应。

to observe/assess 观察

【例 6】

To observe the phenotypic changes of renal tubulo-interstitial cells in human glomerulonephritis.

观察人类肾小球肾炎时肾小管间质细胞发生的表型转化现象。

to analyze/determine/evaluate 分析

【例 7】

To analyze the clinical and pathological characteristics of pancreatic carcinoma in diabetics (DPC) and to explore the relationship between diabetes mellitus and pancreatic carcinoma (PC).

分析胰腺癌合并糖尿病的临床和病理学特征，并探讨糖尿病与胰腺癌之间的关系。

to summarize 总结

【例 8】

To summarize the clinical characteristics of acute pandysautonomia in childhood, to gain a better understanding of the diagnosis and differential diagnosis.

总结儿童急性全自主神经功能不全的临床特征，提高对该病的诊断及鉴别诊断的认识。

注意：描述性英文摘要一般用完整的句子保持语篇照应，结构式摘要则多用动词不定式短语，较少使用完整句子。

2）表达方法（Methods）

医学论文英文摘要中的 Methods 部分旨在提供论文的科学依据，概括研究所用的原理、条件、材料、对象和方法，并提供正误对照说明。总体来说，这部分的内容包括两大层次：研究方案和研究过程；再具体些，还可以包括研究对象和研究方法。这部分的常用句型如下所示：

（1）表示研究过程的持续时间

during/over the past 10 years 近 10 年来

in the past 10 years 过去 10 年中

during/in the period of 2020 to 2024 / during/in the 2020–2024 period

2020—2024 年

from January 2020 to December 2024 / between January 2020 and December 2024

2020 年 1 月—2024 年 12 月

【例】

A retrospective analysis was performed in the Department of Endocrinology Peking Union Medical College Hospital **from October 1981 to June 2019**. Patients with PAI as the first symptom were enrolled. The etiology of PAI was analyzed and the clinical characteristics were also summarized.

回顾性分析 1981 年 10 月—2019 年 6 月北京协和医院内分泌科以 PAI 为首发症状的患者的病例资料，对病因进行分析并总结其临床特点。

（2）表示研究对象（人或实验动物）特征（包括性别、年龄、种族等）及样本量

We assessed... between... and...

我们评估了……和……之间……

【例】

We assessed the association **between** exercise capacity **and** mortality in black (*n* = 6,749; age, 58 + 11 years) and white (*n* = 8,911; age, 60 + 11 years) male veterans with and without cardiovascular disease who successfully completed a treadmill exercise test at the Veterans Affairs Medical Centers in Washington D.C., and Palo Alto, California. Fitness categories were based on peak metabolic equivalents (METs) achieved. Subjects were followed up for all-cause mortality for 7.5 + 5.3 years.

我们评估了黑人（*n* = 6 749；年龄，58 + 11 岁）和白人（*n* = 8 911；年龄，60 + 11 岁）男性退伍军人（无论是否有心血管疾病）的运动能力与死亡率之间的关系，他们在华盛顿特区和加利福尼亚州帕洛阿尔托的退伍军人事务医疗中心成功完成了跑步机运动测试。体能类别是基于所达到的峰值代谢当量。对受试者进行了 7.5 + 5.3 年的全因死亡随访。

（3）检查和手术治疗 / 排除标准及观察

... was done/performed/in/on... patients / ... patients underwent...

对……患者做了……检查 / 手术

【例】

Routine physical examination **was performed on patients**, and criteria were given to patients. Exclusion criteria included comorbid history of epilepsy, < 2 PNES/month, and IQ < 70. The primary outcome was seizure frequency at the end of treatment and at 6-month follow-up. Secondary outcomes included 3 months of seizure freedom at 6-month follow-up.

对患者进行了常规体格检查，并给出了标准。排除标准包括癫痫史，精神性非癫痫发作每月小于两次，智商 < 70。主要观测指标为治疗结束时和 6 个月随访期的发作频率。次级指标包括 6 个月随访期中 3 个月内无癫痫发作。

（4）研究方法

using/employing... / ... was used/employed/applied to do... 用……法（去做）

【例】

Using data from patients hospitalized in a cohort of 890 U.S. hospitals during the period 2012–2017, we generated national case counts for both hospital-onset and community-onset infections caused by methicillin-resistant Staphylococcus aureus (MRSA), vancomycin-resistant enterococcus (VRE), extended-spectrum cephalosporin resistance in Enterobacteriaceae suggestive of extended-spectrum beta-lactamase (ESBL) production, carbapenem-resistant Enterobacteriaceae, carbapenem-resistant acinetobacter species, and MDR pseudomonas aeruginosa.

利用 2012—2017 年美国 890 家医院的住院患者数据，我们对由耐甲氧西林金黄色葡萄球菌、耐万古霉素肠球菌、肠杆菌科中的超广谱头孢菌素耐药性提示产生超广谱 β–内酰胺酶、碳青霉烯类耐药肠杆菌科、碳青霉烯类耐药不动杆菌属和耐多药铜绿假单胞菌等引起的医院发病和社区发病的感染性病例进行了全国统计。

（5）有关剂量的表达

in a dose / each dose 每次剂量

daily dosage / the dosage in a day 每天剂量

the initial dose/dosage 首次剂量

the/a total dose/dosage of 总剂量

【例】

We randomly assigned 48 surgical patients ≥ 65 years of age to receive single intranasal doses of dexmedetomidine or placebo (5:1 ratio) in four sequential dose cohorts: 0.5, 1.0, 1.5, and 2.0 μg/kg. **Each dose** cohort comprised two groups of six subjects: a group of subjects using β-blockers and a group not taking β-blockers. Vital signs and sedation depth (Modified Observer's Assessment of Alertness and Sedation [MOAA/S] and bispectral index) were measured for 2 hours after administration. Blood samples were taken to determine dexmedetomidine plasma concentrations.

我们将 48 名年龄≥ 65 岁的外科患者随机分为 4 个连续剂量组，分别接受右美托咪定或安慰剂（5：1）的单次鼻内给药：0.5、1.0、1.5 和 2.0 微克/千克。每个剂量队列包括两组，每组六名受试者：一组受试者使用 β 受体阻滞剂；另一组不使用 β 受体阻滞剂。给药后 2 个小时测量生命体征和镇静深度（修正的观察者警觉和镇静评估和脑电双频谱指数）。采集血样以测定右美托咪定的血浆浓度。

（6）有关疗效的表达

curative/therapeutic effect / efficacy of the treatment/drug 疗效

good therapeutic / curative effect/result / respond well to 疗效好

criteria to test the efficacy/effectiveness 疗效判断标准

【例】

Criteria to test the efficacy of using antibiotics to treat chronic lymphocytic leukemia.

使用抗生素治疗慢性淋巴细胞白血病疗效判断标准。

3）表达结果（Results）

结果是对实验结果的详细描述，是摘要部分的核心，通常用实验数据说明实验前后的变化。对于结果的书写，作者须凸显研究中的客观资料和重要发现，描述应体现可信度和准确性。英文需用完整句子，谓语动词采用过去时态，研究所用的资料，如百分数、血压等数字采用临床病例书写形式，不必用书面英文表达。

（1）有关结果的表达

The result(s) showed/suggested/indicated/documented that...

结果表明……

【例】

The result showed that the speed of symptom improvement decreased significantly after several acupuncture courses.

结果表明，几个针灸疗程之后，症状改善的速度明显下降。

（2）有关发现的表达

It was found that... / We found that...

（我们）发现……

【例】

We found that the speed of symptom improvement decreased significantly after several acupuncture courses.

我们发现几个针灸疗程之后，症状改善的速度明显下降。

（3）有关增加或减少的表达

increased/decreased by 增加 / 减少

【例】

The data shows that the frequency of heart attack **decreased by** the dose of medicine at the end of treatment.

数据显示，在治疗结束时，心脏病发作的频率随着药物剂量的减少而降低。

（4）有关差异的表达

There was significant/statistical difference between... and...

在……和……之间有显著 / 统计差异。

Significant difference was found...

……具有显著差异 / 发现了显著差异。

【例】

There was significant difference between the SERS (Side Effects Rating Scale) scores of two groups ($P < 0.05$); the control group had more adverse reactions, and the score would be increased with the extension of treatment time.

两组副作用评定量表评分差异有统计学意义（$P < 0.05$）；对照组不良反应较多，随着治疗时间的延长，副作用评定量表评分增加。

4）表达结论（Conclusion）

结论是作者对研究结果的综合分析，通常比较简短，用一两句话概括研究结果、局限性和未来展望。

注意：若结论具有普遍性，英文动词用一般现在时；若结论不具备普遍性，英文动词用一般过去时。

（1）suggest

The authors suggest that... / It is suggested that...

作者建议 / 认为……

The data obtained suggest that...

所获得的资料表明……

【例】

Together **these data suggest that** C4 activation is critical for initiating renal flare while C3 activation is involved in the actual tissue damage, and that these effects are influenced by genetic variability in complement activation and regulation.

这些数据表明，C4 的激活对肾炎发作起重要作用，而 C3 的激活则导致组织损伤，这些作用都受到了补体激活与调节的遗传变异的影响。

（2）conclude/conclusion

Our conclusion is that... / We conclude that...

我们的结论是……

From this we can conclude that...

由此可得出以下结论……

【例】

Our conclusion is that C4 activation is critical for initiating renal flare while C3 activation is involved in the actual tissue damage, and that these effects are influenced by genetic variability in complement activation and regulation.

我们的结论是，C4 的激活对肾炎发作起重要作用，而 C3 的激活则导致组织损伤，这些作用都受到了补体激活与调节的遗传变异的影响。

（3）show/indicate

The result/data shows...

结果 / 数据显示……

The study indicates that...

研究表明……

【例】

The study indicates that C4 activation is critical for initiating renal flare while C3 activation is involved in the actual tissue damage, and that these effects are influenced by genetic variability in complement activation and regulation.

研究表明，C4 的激活对肾炎发作起重要作用，而 C3 的激活则导致组织损伤，这些作用都受到了补体激活与调节的遗传变异的影响。

（4）illustrate/demonstrate/confirm

This case illustrates that...

本例说明……

These results demonstrate that...

这些结果证明 / 显示……

【例】

This case illustrates that C4 activation is critical for initiating renal flare while C3 activation is involved in the actual tissue damage, and that these effects are influenced by genetic variability in complement activation and regulation.

本例说明，C4 的激活对肾炎发作起重要作用，而 C3 的激活则导致组织损伤，这些作用都受到了补体激活与调节的遗传变异的影响。

（5）feel/believe/think/consider

We feel/believe think/consider that...

我们认为……

We strongly believe that...

我们深信……

【例】

We strongly believe that C4 activation is critical for initiating renal flare while C3 activation is involved in the actual tissue damage, and that these effects are influenced by genetic variability in complement activation and regulation.

我们深信，C4 的激活对肾炎发作起重要作用，而 C3 的激活则导致组织损伤，这些作用都受到了补体激活与调节的遗传变异的影响。

（6）point out

It is pointed out that...

指出……

【例】

It is pointed out that C4 activation is critical for initiating renal flare while C3 activation is involved in the actual tissue damage, and that these effects are influenced by genetic variability in complement activation and regulation.

研究指出，C4 的激活对肾炎发作起重要作用，而 C3 的激活则导致组织损伤，这些作用都受到了补体激活与调节的遗传变异的影响。

（7）propose/recommend

The authors propose that...

作者提出……

It is proposed that...

提出……

【例】

The authors propose that C4 activation is critical for initiating renal flare while C3 activation is involved in the actual tissue damage, and that these effects are influenced by genetic variability in complement activation and regulation.

作者提出，C4 的激活对肾炎发作起重要作用，而 C3 的激活则导致组织损伤，这些作用都受到了补体激活与调节的遗传变异的影响。

（8）support

These results strongly support that...

这些结果有力地支持……

【例】

These results strongly support that C4 activation is critical for initiating renal flare while C3 activation is involved in the actual tissue damage, and that these effects are influenced by genetic variability in complement activation and regulation.

这些结果有力地支持了 C4 的激活对肾炎发作起重要作用，而 C3 的激活则导致组织损伤，这些作用都受到了补体激活与调节的遗传变异的影响。

（9）significance

be of great/some significance in/of/to 具有……意义

【例】

Imaging examination **is of great importance in** the diagnosis of patients with suspected clinical cases, the investigation of asymptomatic infections and family clustering, the judgment of patient recovery, rediagnosis after disease recurrence, and prognosis prediction.

影像学检查对临床疑似病例患者的诊断、无症状感染者与家族聚集的调查、患者康复判断、疾病复发后再诊断、预后预测具有重要意义。

2. 摘要的语言时态特点

摘要的目的部分主要介绍一般性资料、现象或普遍事实，多使用一般现在时；用 however、but、yet、few、little、no 等指出过去研究的不足并引出作者的研究问题时，使用现在完成时；叙述本人或他人近期的工作时，采用过去时。方法部分常用一般过去时，表示回顾性叙述，且多用被动语态。结果部分是回顾性陈述，除描述性说明外，一般用过去时态。撰写结论部分时，如果结论具有普遍性，用一般现在时；如果结论仅是一种可能性或只表示当时的研究结果和研究范围，则用一般过去时。

7.3 关键词（Keywords）

7.3.1 关键词的定义

关键词也称索引词、主题词，是文献搜索的重要依据，必须能表达论文的主题及中心内容，一般选 3 ~ 5 个词或短语；常用名词、名词短语或者复合词，尽量避免使用动词、形容词、缩略语等。

7.3.2 关键词的书写格式

关于关键词的书写格式，不同的期刊要求略有不同。有的期刊排列关键词用分号隔开，最末一个词后不加符号；各关键词之间也可不用标点符号。多数医学期刊要求每个关键词的首字母大写，有的要求字母全部大写。多数医学期刊用 Keywords、Key Words，也有医学期刊用 MeSH、Subjective Words/Headings 等。因此，作者向某杂志投稿时，应事先了解其编写要求。

7.3.3 关键词的标引

关键词列举不当，是作者容易犯的错误，作者应避免关键词遗漏、术语表达或写作概念错误、重复标引关键词、关键词标引顺序不当、使用过时的医学概念，以及注意英美英语的差异问题等。

注意：在使用规范术语时，我们应尽量选用由中国医学科学院医学信息研究所翻译出版的《医学文献索引》（*Index Medicus*，*IM*）中的《医学主题词表》（*Medical Subject Headings*，*MeSH*）和中国中医研究院图书情报研究所编制的中医药主题词表中所列的词，若未收录在以上文献中，我们则可以直接将该新术语作为关键词。

7.4 署名与工作单位（Signature and Work Unit）

7.4.1 署名

一般情况下，国内外医学期刊要求在标题下写上作者的名字、学位和工作单位。2013 年 8 月发布的《学术研究实施与报告和医学期刊编辑与发表的推荐规范》（*Recommendations for the Conduct, Reporting, Editing, and Publication of Scholarly Work in Medical Journals*），简称《ICMJE 推荐规范》，从各方面明确规定了作者的定义，同时指出须同时满足四个方面的条件才能成为作者。

一般须根据作者对研究工作和论文撰写的贡献大小来安排署名，一旦确定，不可随意改动。通常情况下，除通讯作者外，贡献越大，排名越靠前。多数期刊要求作者在投稿时写明每一位作者在该研究中的具体贡献。很多情况下，通讯作者和第一作者是同一个人。

署名应真实，用全名。人名拼音拼写规则主要遵循《中国人名汉语拼音字母拼写规则》（标准号：GB/T 28039—2011），姓和名分开写，而双姓（如司马、欧阳）和双名不可分开写，姓和名的首字母大写；此外，还应参考拟投期刊的要求。作者应尽量采用相对固定的署名方式，以增强文献检索和论文引用的准确性。

7.4.2 作者学位

为了避免姓名相同造成文献混乱，有的国外医学期刊要求姓名之后附有学位、职称及作为国际享有较高声誉的某学会会员的身份缩写。国内医学期刊一般不刊出作者学位。常见的学位如下所示：

- M.B. (MB) = Bachelor of Medicine 医学学士
- M.M. (MM) = Master of Medicine 医学硕士
- M.D. (MD) = Doctor of Medicine 医学博士
- Ph.D. (PhD) = Doctor of Philosophy 博士 / 哲学博士

7.4.3 作者单位

工作单位及属地是指作者所属工作机构及机构所在地，是期刊编辑部或读者与作者直接联系的重要信息源，国内外医学期刊对工作单位的排列顺序和排版位置都有一定的格式要求。

1. 单位常用词

在英文中，工作单位的排列顺序应合乎英文表达的规范。小的单位单元常涉及如下常用词：

- 部门 / 科 / 处：division
- 科 / 系：department
- 研究所 / 学院：institute
- 处 / 中心：center
- 部门 / 处 / 组：section
- 实验室：laboratory
- 部门 / 处：branch

其中，division、section 和 branch 意义比较接近，基本可以通用。

【例】

Division of Newborn Medicine, Department of Pediatrics, the Mount Sinai School of Medicine, New York, NY, U.S.

美国纽约西奈山医学院儿科学系新生儿科

2. 单位排列顺序

在国外医学期刊的论文中，单位名称的排列顺序大致有以下三种：

（1）小单位在前，大单位在后，如科、院、校、市、州、省、国。

【例】

Division of Gastroenterology, Department of Medicine, University of Texas Medical School, Houston, Texas, U.S.

美国得克萨斯州休斯敦市得克萨斯大学医学院医学系胃肠科

（2）大单位在前，小单位在后。

【例】

University of Chicago, Department of Surgery

芝加哥大学外科学系

（3）前两种排列顺序的混合型。

【例】

Department of Medicine Division of Digestive Diseases, University of Mississippi Medical Center, Jackson, Mississippi

密西西比州杰克逊市密西西比大学医学中心内科消化病组

在国内医学期刊的英文摘要中，单位名称的排列通常采用小单位在前，大单位在后的形式。

3. 单位排版位置

在国外医学杂志刊登的论文中，常见的工作单位的编排位置有两种：①用斜体字直接排列在作者姓名之下；②标题下只写作者姓名，单位名称置于论文首页下方的脚注中，这时，工作单位名称前一般要用介词 from。目前，很多国外医学期刊采用第二种署名格式。

国内医学学术期刊常见的排版有四种：①工作单位一般置于作者姓名下方，并加邮政编码。②工作单位名称用斜体字排在姓名之后，而英文版则将工作单位名称以脚注形式置于论文首页右下角。③若作者来自不同单位，则将工作单位分别排在作者姓名之下。④作者来自不同单位的另一种表达方式是在作者姓名之后右上角与单位名称之前左上角分别用相同的符号，如加星号或阿拉伯数字。工作单位名称之前省略介词 from。具体还应参考出版期刊的要求而定。

4. 单位翻译问题

医学论文写作发表的最终目的是学术交流。这种交流不局限于国内，还包括国际交流，因此医学论文各部分尤其是署名及工作单位的翻译很重要。我国单位名称多且较复杂，所以无法统一翻译标准，这也势必导致英译的单位名称五花八门。书写单位名称时，应注意以下几点：① 采用作者单位已有的译名。② 高等学校、医疗单位、研究所等应具体到二级或三级机构。③ 采用汉语拼音拼写名称时，要按《汉语拼音正词法基本规则》(标准号: GB/T 16159—2012)规范拼写。④ 单位所在区域邮政编码需认真核实,防止造成邮件分拣过程出现差错,导致邮件投递延误。⑤ 对于基层医疗机构,虽然有邮政编码可以确认单位所在地,但由于中国的行政区划分与国外存在一定的差异,单位名称与地址应尽可能详尽,如中国某省某县某乡某卫生所的表达方式为"XXX Clinic, XXX Country (+ 邮编), XXX County, XXX Province, China"。

Exercises

Exercise I　Change the following titles into the ones with proper subtitles.

1. 30 Years' Experience with Hysterectomy for Benign Conditions
2. Orphan Disease or Persistent Problem in Bronchiectasis in Children
3. Evidence-Based Medicine Is a New Approach to Teaching the Practice of Medicine

Exercise II　Decide which type the following titles belong to.

1. Orphan Disease or Persistent Problem in Bronchiectasis in Children
2. Thyroid Carcinoma Induced by Irradiation for Hodgkin's Disease
3. On the Influence of Technology in Modern Society
4. Factors that Predict Outcome of Abdominal Operations in Patients with Advanced Cirrhosis
5. Is Autophagy in Cell Death an Innocent Convict?

Exercise III　Translate the following titles into Chinese or English.

1. 本文旨在研究肾移植患者的并发症。
2. 请采用合理的句型格式将以下"目的"句译为英文或中文。
3. 研究初发性急性白血病的疗效及影响因素。
4. BP was measured twice by trained observers using a standard mercury sphygmomanometer after the subject had been seated for at least five minutes.
5. All samples have been frozen at –20℃ until tasted by conventional ELISA.
6. This result indicated that the speed of symptom improvement decreased significantly after several acupuncture courses.
7. Compared with before the treatment, the scores on menstrual color and quantity soreness and weakness of waist and knee, and breast swelling pain were decreased in both groups after treatment ($P < 0.05$).

8. In summary, our findings elucidated the potential mechanism of Baoyuan decoction on cardio-protection, and further explained its traditional efficacy in the molecular level.

9. However, there was potential bias in the included studies, so the conclusion still needed further high quality randomized controlled trials to improve the evidence level.

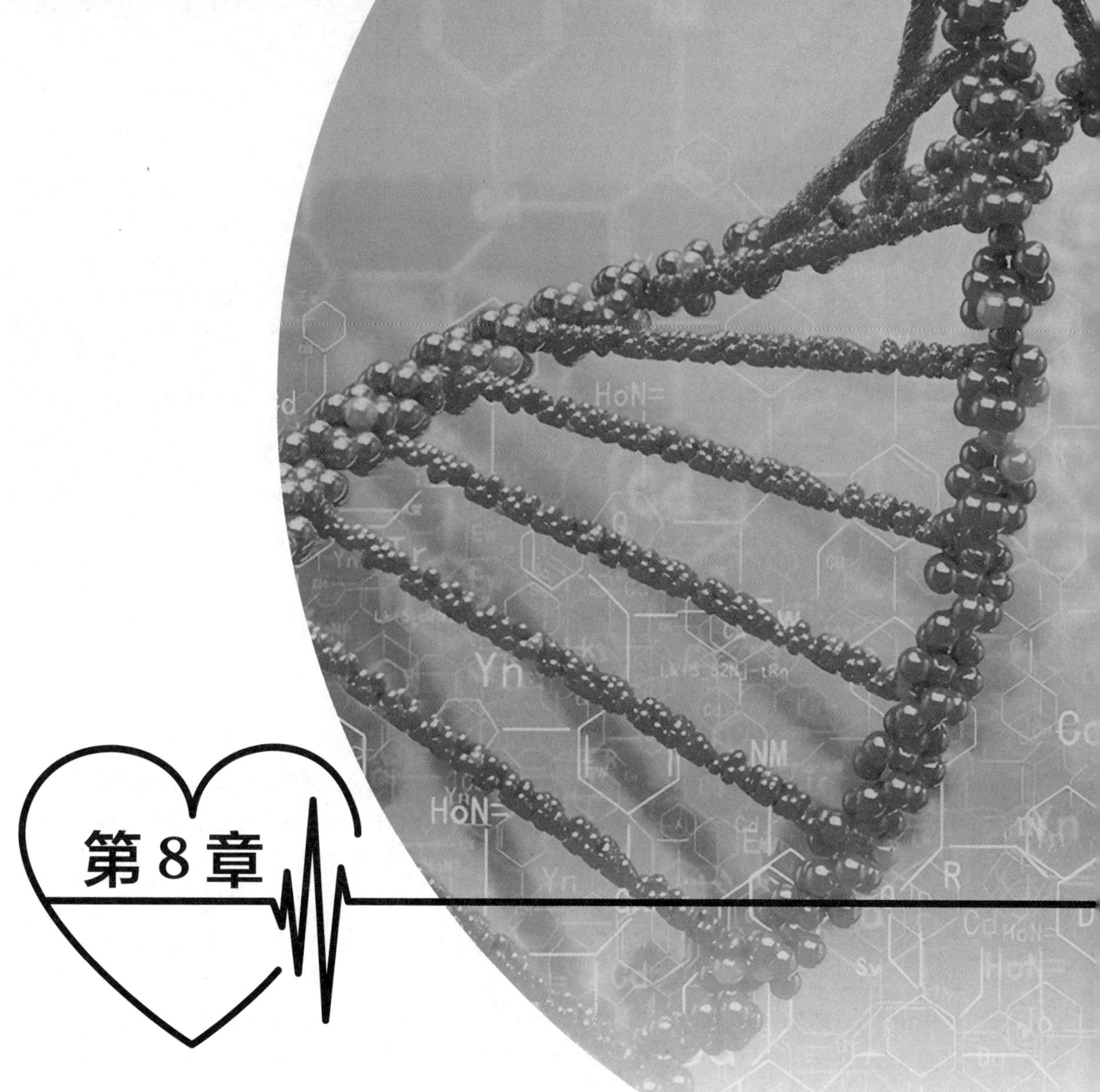

第 8 章

医学研究论文 I（Medical Research Papers I）

Medicines are not meant to live on.

不能靠药物度日。

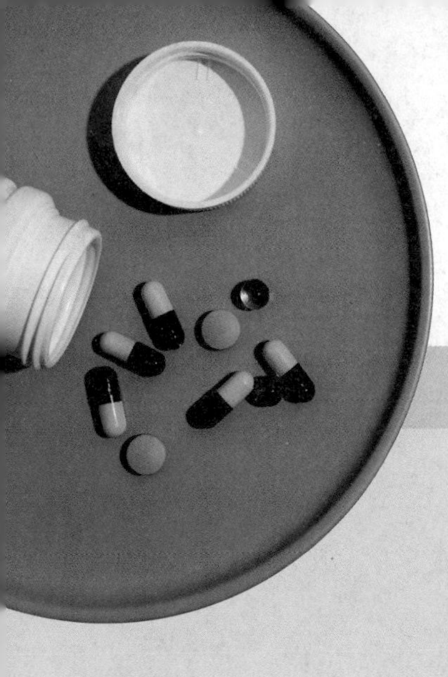

Warm-up

1. Think of yourself as a reader for a moment. What kind of papers do you like to read?

2. Do you know the four parts of the text of a biomedical research paper?

国际医学期刊编辑委员会（International Committee of Medical Journal Editors，ICMJE）公布的《生物医学期刊投稿的统一要求》（Uniform Requirements for Manuscripts Submitted to Biomedical Journals）（温哥华格式）和国内颁布的《科学技术报告、学位论文和学术论文的编写格式》，都对医学论文的格式、内容和投稿做了具体的规定。医学英语论文主要由标题（Title）、作者（Authorship）、摘要与关键词（Abstract and Keywords）、引言（Introduction）、材料与方法（Materials and Methods）、结果（Results）、讨论（Discussion）、致谢（Acknowledgements）和参考文献（References）九部分组成。本章主要介绍医学英语论文正文部分的结构与要求。

8.1 引言（Introduction）

8.1.1 引言部分的内容与写法

引言也称前言、导言或序言，是一篇论文正文的开始部分，简要介绍研究的背景和理由，说明研究的内容和目的，要点如下：

（1）说明本研究项目的背景，国内外同类课题的研究现状、进展及尚待解决的问题；

（2）回顾与本研究有关的论文和著作及文献资料的来源（注明文献号）和收集方法；

（3）介绍本研究的起止日期、采用的方法、主要结果、意义或必要性；

（4）介绍作者对本研究已发表的论文及其结论；

（5）介绍本研究的内容和目的、实验设计、预期结果及价值。

在实际写作过程中，作者可根据需要对上述内容有所取舍。引言的写作顺序通常是先介绍本研究的背景，然后说明研究的总体范围、进展（如已有发现、报告或研究），最后提出研究意义和目的。阐述研究目的时，应简明扼要，一般用一两个句子加以概括即可。引言一般为 200 ~ 300 词。

8.1.2 常用句型和时态

（1）表示已知信息，常用一般现在时或现在完成时，如：

... is known to...

... is widely used in...

... has been reported that...

... has been proved that...

... has long been successfully applied for...

（2）表示未知信息，常用一般现在时或现在完成时，如：

... is unclear.

... is unknown.

... has not been established.

... has not been determined.

... remains an important unsolved problem.

（3）表示不确定性，常用情态动词（猜测性用法）或某些形容词，如：

... might reduce...

... may have an effect on...

... could damage...

... remain controversial...

... is still uncertain...

（4）表示研究的内容和目的，常用一般过去时，如：

We hypothesized that...

In this study we asked whether...

We designed a prospective trial to test whether...

The purpose of this study was to determine whether...

The current study was, therefore, designed to determine whether...

8.1.3 示例

下面是一篇题为“Effect of Alkalosis on Hypoxia-induced Pulmonary Vasoconstriction in Lungs from Newborn Rabbits”（《碱中毒对缺氧所致新生兔肺血管收缩的影响》）的论文的引言部分：

Alkalosis, produced primarily by mechanical hyperventilation, is widely used in the treatment of newborns who have the syndrome of persistent pulmonary hypertension. (已知信息) Although mechanical hyperventilation is often clinically effective in the treatment of these infants, it is not clear whether the clinical improvements during mechanical hyperventilation are due to the alkalosis resulting from the therapy. (未知信息) The results of the few studies of the effect of alkalosis on hypoxia-induced pulmonary vasoconstriction in lungs of newborn animals have been variable. Alkalosis has been shown either to reduce or to have no effect on constriction of the neonatal pulmonary circulation in response to alveolar hypoxia. (已知信息) These variable results may have been caused by the different sequences in which the lungs were exposed to hypoxia and alkalosis. (不确定性) If alkalosis does reduce hypoxia-induced pulmonary vasoconstriction, some of its harmful effects might be avoided by using metabolic instead of mechanical (respiratory) alkalosis. (研究必要性)

In this study, we asked whether or not alkalosis reduces constriction of the neonatal pulmonary circulation in response to hypoxia and whether metabolic alkalosis is as effective as respiratory alkalosis. To answer these questions, we measured the vasoconstrictive responses of isolated, perfused lungs from newborn rabbits to respiratory or metabolic alkalosis and hypoxia in three sequences: alkalosis before, during, and after alveolar hypoxia. (研究的内容和目的)

碱中毒主要由过度机械通气引起，广泛用于治疗新生儿持续性肺动脉高压综合征。虽然过度机械通气在这些婴儿的治疗中通常是有临床效果的，但目前尚不清楚过度机械通气期间的临床改善是否由治疗引起的碱中毒所致。碱中毒对新生动物肺缺氧引起的肺血管收缩的影响的少数研究结果是可变的。已有研究表明，碱中毒可以减少或不影响肺泡缺氧引起的新生儿肺循环收缩。这些不同的结果可能是由于肺暴露于缺氧和碱中毒的不同顺序造成的。如果碱中毒确实能减轻缺氧引起的肺血管收缩，用代谢性碱中毒代替机械性（呼吸性）碱中毒可避免其某些不良影响。

在这项研究中，我们询问碱中毒是否会减少新生儿缺氧时肺循环的收缩，以及代谢性碱中毒是否与呼吸性碱中毒一样有效。为了回答这些问题，我们测量了新生兔离体灌流肺对呼吸性或代谢性碱中毒和缺氧的血管收缩反应，分为三个序列：肺泡缺氧之前、期间和之后的碱中毒。

这个引言由两个自然段组成：第一段介绍了有关该课题的研究现状，包括已取得的进展和尚未阐明的问题；第二段说明了该研究的内容。

8.2 材料与方法（Materials and Methods）

8.2.1 材料与方法的内容与写法

材料与方法是临床试验、实验研究和现场调查的手段，是判断论文科学性、创新性的主要依据，是研究结果的基础部分，故应具体而真实地说明研究如何设计、研究所使用的材料和方法，以供他人理解、学习和重复验证。

作者可根据具体的论文类型选用如下标题：对象和方法（Patients/Participants/Subjects and Methods）、病例和方法（Cases and Methods）、设计与方法（Design and Methods）、病例报告（Case Reports）、临床资料（Clinical Information）、手术方法（Methods of Operation）、调查方法（Methods of Investigation）、测量方法（Methods of Measurement）等。

在结构式摘要中，论文的材料与方法可简称为方法（Methods）。

材料与方法一般包含四个部分：研究设计（study design）、研究对象（study subjects）、测量方法（methods of measurement）、统计分析（statistic analysis）。

1. 研究设计

这部分须包括研究对象的随机分组（对照组与治疗组）、选择标准、回顾、前瞻、临床、动物、实验、随访、人群、流行病等研究性质；必要时，作者还要说明处理方式，包括治疗方法、手术方法、仪器、药物（注明生产单位、商标、出厂日期及批号等）。

【例】

在“Hypertension Is Associated with Osteoporosis: A Case-Control Study in Chinese Postmenopausal Women”（《高血压与骨质疏松有关：中国绝经后女性的病例对照研究》）这篇论文中，研究设计是通过设置研究组和对照组来确定的。

In total, 2,873 participants completed the baseline survey from January 2007 to October 2019, and 2,039 were included in this retrospective study. We divided all subjects into an osteoporosis group and a non-osteoporosis group based on their bone mineral density (BMD). Dual-energy X-ray absorptiometry (DXA) was used to examine BMD. The general information came from the questionnaire survey. Cardiovascular diseases were defined by asking participants at the first visit and checking relevant medical records if they had suffered from hypertension, coronary heart disease, or cerebral infarction.

2007 年 1 月至 2019 年 10 月，共有 2 873 名参与者完成了基线调查，其中 2 039 名参与者被纳入本次回顾性研究。我们根据骨密度将所有受试者分为骨质疏松症组和非骨质疏松症组，采用双能 X 射线吸收测定法检测骨密度。一般信息来自问卷调查。心血管疾病是通过在第一次就诊时询问参与者并检查他们是否患有高血压、冠心病或脑梗死的相关病历来确定的。

2. 研究对象

研究对象一般指患者、受试者、健康志愿者及动物，要经过严格的筛选，尽量减少因个体差异而引起的不准确因素。因此，研究对象应尽可能具有共性，具体要求如下：

（1）以人为研究对象，应注明性别、年龄、体重、职业、病程、病因、病情、生理状态、化验室检查、特殊检查、既往用药史、治疗史、分组情况、诊断标准、分型标准及其他区别特性。

（2）若受试对象为实验动物，要说明实验动物的种类、数量、来源、品系、年龄、身长、性别、体重、健康状况及分组标准等。

（3）研究对象若是微生物，要标明种系、菌株、血清类型及其他特征。

（4）实验报告中涉及人时，应明确实验过程是否符合社会事业机构或地区性的人体实验委员会制定的伦理道德标准或《赫尔辛基宣言》（*The Declaration of Helsinki*）；不可使用患者的真实姓名、缩写名及医院代码。

（5）实验报告中涉及实验动物时，应说明是否符合相关机构、国家研究委员会或者国家法律关于实验室动物的管理与使用准则。

在临床研究中，论文多采用回顾性形式，应尽量增加观察的病例数。

【例】

下面是"Behavioral and Pharmacological Therapies for Late-Life Insomnia: A Randomized Controlled Trial"（《老年失眠的行为和药物治疗：随机对照试验》）这篇论文中关于研究对象的表述：

This retrospective study was carried out from January 2007 to October 2019 with participants from Fuzhou, capital of Fujian Province. All participants were investigated in the Department of Osteoporosis of the Fujian Academy of Chinese Medical Sciences. The 2,873 participants aged between 41 and 90 accepted the questionnaire survey, and 2,039 natural postmenopausal women who met the criteria were included in this study.

All subjects could provide complete medical records and sign informed consent independently. All participants were excluded if they had hyperparathyroidism, diabetes, rheumatoid arthritis, or other endocrine and immune diseases that affect bone metabolism. Patients with severe liver, kidney, or haematopoietic diseases and malignant tumors were also excluded. Further, none of the subjects had received osteoporosis treatment or other known drugs that affect bone metabolism. No potential subjects had missing key data. Written consent was necessary for all participants.

这项回顾性研究于 2007 年 1 月至 2019 年 10 月进行，参与者来自福建省省会福州。所有参与者均在福建省中医药科学院骨质疏松症科接受调查。2 873 名年龄在 41 岁至 90 岁的参与者接受了问卷调查，符合标准的 2 039 名自然绝经后的女性被纳入本研究。

所有受试者均能提供完整的病历并独立签署知情同意书。所有患有甲状旁腺功能亢进症、糖尿病、类风湿性关节炎或其他影响骨代谢的内分泌和免疫疾病的参与者均被排除在外。患有严重肝、肾或造血系统疾病和恶性肿瘤的患者也被排除在外。此外，没有受试者接受过骨质疏松症治疗或其他影响骨代谢的已知药物。没有潜在受试者缺少关键数据。所有参与者都需要书面同意。

3. 测量方法

凡属作者创新的实验设计、临床观察、手术方法、治疗效果、实验步骤等都要做出详细说明，以便同行能重复这个实验。若有新的或实质性改进的方法，则要说明采用这类方法的理由，并讲述改进的创新部分；若属临床方面资料，应介绍治疗方法和措施，包括确切地说明所使用药物的剂型和剂量、给药途径和疗程、有无其他药物同时使用；若为作者发明创造，如实验仪器，应在不违反保密原则、不影响专利权的前提下，全面介绍其结构、性能、原理、用途、使用方法，必要时，可附结构图或设计图；若为前人所用过或公知公认的方法，只写明其方法名称即可；引用他人的方法时，应注明文献和出处，但无须详细介绍。

【例】

The data required for the study came from the questionnaire survey. General information, such as age, height, weight, blood pressure, menarche age, menopausal age, past medical history, and personal lifestyle, was collected and carefully filled in the unified form by trained physicians. Height and weight were measured without shoes, and the body mass index (BMI) was calculated. Before blood pressure measurement, participants needed to rest quietly for at least five minutes, empty their bladders, and not take any drugs. The data used were the average of two measurements.

Bone Mineral Density Measurement

Dual-energy X-ray absorptiometry (DXA) (Discovery W, Hologic Inc., U.S.) was used to measure BMD of the lumbar spine and left femoral neck. The T score was calculated according to the reference range of the instrument manufacturer. The inspection was performed daily by the same professional physician. The coefficient of variation (CV) for repeated measurements was approximately 1.0%.

研究所需数据来自问卷调查。收集一般信息，如年龄、身高、体重、血压、初潮年龄、绝经年龄、既往病史和个人生活方式，并由训练有素的医生仔细填写在统一的表格中。脱鞋测量身高和体重，并计算身体质量指数。测量血压前，参与者需要安静休息至少五分钟，排空膀胱，不服用任何药物。使用的数据是两次测量的平均值。

骨密度测量

双能 X 射线骨密度仪（Discovery W, Hologic Inc., U.S.）用于测量腰椎和左股骨颈的骨密度。T 值是根据仪器制造商的参考范围计算的。每天由同一位专业医师进行检查。重复测量的变异系数约为 1.0%。

4. 统计分析

《生物医学期刊投稿的统一要求》给出如下建议：①有关统计学方法的描述应尽可能详尽，以保证读者能够通过原始数据核实所报告的结果。②如有可能，应对结果进行量化，并提供测定误差或不确定性（如可信区间的合适指标）。③应避免仅仅依靠统计学的假定性检验，如只有 *P* 值就不能体现重要的量化信息。④对实验对象的可靠性、随机化的具体细节、观察方法、盲法对照的可靠程度、处理措施引起的并发症、观察例数、未能观察的具体情况（如临床试验中因各种原因而终止观察）等均应做详细描述。⑤有关实验设计和统计学方法的参考文献应尽可能引用标准著作（注明所在页码），而不引用那些首先报告有关实验设计或方法的文献。⑥指出所有已采用的计算通用程度。⑦不要随意使用统计学中的一些专业术语，如随机（表示随机化设计）、正常、显著、相关、样本等。⑧注明统计学术语、缩略语和符号。

注意：在处理数据时，应避免统计方法错误，以保证论文的科学性和可信度。

【例】

EpiData 2 (The EpiData Association, Odense M, Denmark) was used to enter and proofread data repeatedly, and SPSS 23.0 (IBM, Inc., New York, U.S.) software was used to conduct all analyses. The results are expressed as the average standard deviation or quantity (percentage). We used the independent samples t-test or Mann-Whitney U-test according to whether the continuous variables conformed to the normal distribution. The Pearson chi-square test was used to measure the difference in frequency. Logistic regression analysis was confirmed with osteoporosis as a dependent variable to investigate the factors affecting osteoporosis. First, the independent variables were screened. Univariate regression analysis was used to exclude non-statistically significant variables ($P > 0.05$) and eliminate the mediator variables. Multicollinearity was assessed using stepwise regression. For continuous variables, the linear condition was assessed. The –2 log-likelihood ratio was used to test the overall significance of the model. The Hosmer-Lemshow test evaluated the model's goodness-of-fit. All statistical hypothesis tests were two-sided and performed at the 0.05 significance level.

将 EpiData 2（The EpiData Association, Odense M, Denmark）用于重复输入和校对数据，并使用 SPSS 23.0（IBM, Inc., New York, U.S.）软件进行所有分析。结果以平均标准偏差或数量（百分比）表示。根据连续变量是否符合正态分布，我们使用独立样本 t 检验或 Mann-Whitney U 检验。Pearson 卡方检验用于测量频率差异。以骨质疏松症为因变量进行逻辑回归分析，探讨影响骨质疏松症的因素。首先，筛选自变量。单变量回归分析用于排除非统计显著变量（$P > 0.05$）并消除中介变量。使用逐步回归评估多重共线性。对于连续变量，评估线性条件。–2 对数似然比用于检验模型的整体显著性。Hosmer-Lemshow 检验评估了模型的拟合优度。所有统计假设检验都是双侧的，并在 0.05 显著性水平下进行。

8.2.2 常用表达

1）选择研究对象

（1）Inclusion/Entry/Exclusion criteria were/included...

纳入 / 入组 / 排除标准为 / 包括……

（2）Selection was based on... / ... were selected based on...

选择是基于……

（3）The major criteria for inclusion in the study were...

纳入研究的主要标准是……

（4）... were entered into / recruited from / selected from / enrolled at...

……从……进入 / 招募 / 选拔 / 注册……

（5）... were excluded from the study/participation.

……被排除在该研究 / 参与之外。

2）表示研究对象分组

（1）... were divided/grouped/stratified/classified/categorized/assigned/randomized into...

……被分成 / 分组 / 分层 / 分类 / 分配 / 随机分到……

（2）... were randomly allocated to... (based on...)

……被随机分配到……（基于……）

3）表示材料来源

（1）... was (obtained) from...

……来源于……

（2）... was provided by...

……由……提供……

（3）... was purchased from...

……购自……

（4）... was donated by / a donation from / a gift from...

……是……捐赠的 / 送的礼物。

4）表示借鉴他人的实验方法

（1）... was isolated/separated by the procedure/technique of...

……被……方法 / 技术分离出来。

（2）... was prepared / carried out according to the method described by...

……是根据……所描述的方法制备 / 进行的。

（3）... was determined by / measured with...

……是由……决定 / 测量的……

5）表示诊断和治疗

（1）... was diagnosed by / diagnostic of...

……被诊断为……

（2）... was diagnosed as/with... (according to / on the basis of...)

……被诊断为……（根据……）

（3）Diagnosis of... was confirmed/made/established.

……的诊断已确认 / 制定 / 确立。

（4）... was misdiagnosed as / mistaken for...

……被误诊为……

（5）... be treated by...

……被……治疗。

（6）... was on... therapy.

……是在……治疗。

（7）... was referred/transferred to...

……被转介 / 调到……

8.3 结果（Results）

8.3.1 结果部分的内容与写法

结果部分是论文的核心、结论的依据，表明该研究的价值，也介绍研究、实验、调查所获得的客观结果，但不包括作者对结果的评述。结果应是建立在数字和分析基础上的信息。写作时，作者应注意以下几点：

（1）结果部分的主要信息就是实验结果，只报告与引言中所提问题相关的结果，既包括支持假设的结果，也包括不支持假设的结果；既包括实验组的结果，也包括对照组的结果。

（2）除报告数据外，作者还要给出有关变化幅度的一般性概念或用百分比表示变化；数据必须准确，且具有内在一致性。

（3）介绍结果时，作者一般不采用简单罗列全部结果的方法，可根据不同情况分层次叙述，如在大段落前设小标题，小标题之下再设分标题。在段落内，作者应按重要性组织资料，最重要的是结果，因此应把结果置于每段段首，把诸如与对照结果、方法、图表、引文和数据相关的辅助性句子放在次要位置。

（4）研究过程难免会出现某些偏差、误差甚至失败的情况，作者也应对此加以说明，一般是将此类说明放在结果的最后部分，把原因分析放在讨论部分。

（5）除了用文字以外，作者还常采用表图叙述的形式表达结果。表注和图注要尽可能详细、具体。表和图内的数据必须与正文相符，若数据已在表或图中呈现，作者便不用在正文中重复表和图的引用，只需在陈述结果的句子后面以括号的方式引用。表和图的内容一般包括两部分——表和图的获得方法，以及对表和图中的数据、图形、符号等做出解释性说明。

【例】

Results

Characteristics of Subjects in the Osteoporosis Group and the Non-Osteoporosis Group

After excluding 834 participants who did not meet the criteria, 2,039 subjects were included in the study. Among these 834 people, 64 were not menopausal, 393 were artificial menopausal, and the rest had other diseases that affect bone metabolism. There were 678 subjects in the osteoporosis group and 1,361 subjects in the non-osteoporosis group. The age of the osteoporosis group was between 47 and 90, and the non-osteoporosis group was between 45 and 85. Statistically, the age and menarche age of subjects who suffered from osteoporosis were significantly older than those who did not, and the menopausal age was more advanced. They also had a lower height and lighter weight ($P < 0.001$). In addition, the BMD of the osteoporosis group was significantly lower than the that of the non-osteoporosis group ($P < 0.001$) (Table 8.1).

Table 8.1 Characteristics of subjects in the osteoporosis group and the non-osteoporosis group (mean ± SD)

Factors	Total (*n* = 2,039)	Osteoporosis (*n* = 678)	Non-Osteoporosis (*n* = 1,361)	*P*
Age (years)	62.56 ± 6.67	64.29 ± 6.71	61.70 ± 6.49	< 0.001[a]
Height (m)	1.59 ± 0.05	1.55 ± 0.05	1.56 ± 0.05	< 0.001[a]
Weight (kg)	57.43 ± 8.39	56.10 ± 8.10	58.08 ± 8.46	< 0.001[a]
BMI (kg/m^2)	23.63 ± 3.10	23.41 ± 3.06	23.74 ± 3.12	0.023[a]
Menarche age (years)	15.39 ± 2.00	15.56 ± 2.10	15.31 ± 1.95	0.021[a]
Menopause age (years)	50.33 ± 3.33	50.10 ± 3.40	50.44 ± 3.29	0.036[a]
Lumbar spine BMD (g/cm^3)	0.77 ± 0.15	0.65 ± 0.08	0.83 ± 0.13	< 0.001[a]
Femoral neck BMD (g/cm^3)	0.73 ± 0.14	0.66 ± 0.14	0.77 ± 0.12	< 0.001[a]

Abbreviations: *BMI = body mass index, BMD = bone mineral density, SD = standard deviation.*

Comparison of Influencing Factors Between the Osteoporosis Group and the Non-Osteoporosis Group

Comparing the influencing factors between the two groups indicated that patients in the osteoporosis group had a higher prevalence of hypertension and coronary heart disease ($P < 0.05$). Besides, the proportion of subjects who drank tea and milk were relatively higher in the osteoporosis group ($P < 0.05$) (Table 8.2).

Table 8.2 Comparison of influencing factors between the osteoporosis group and the non-osteoporosis group (%)

Factors	Total	Osteoporosis	Non-Osteoporosis	*P*
N (%)	2,039 (100)	678 (33.25)	1,361 (66.75)	NA
Drinking coffee, *n* (%)	51 (2.50)	20 (2.95)	31 (2.28)	0.360[a]
Drinking tea, *n* (%)	196 (9.61)	79 (11.65)	117 (8.60)	0.027[a]
Drinking milk, *n* (%)	633 (31.04)	276 (40.71)	357 (26.23)	< 0.001[a]
Hypertension, *n* (%)	359 (17.61)	151 (22.27)	208 (15.28)	< 0.001[a]
Coronary heart disease, *n* (%)	104 (5.10)	50 (7.37)	54 (3.97)	0.001[a]
Cerebral infarction, *n* (%)	22 (1.08)	9 (1.33)	13 (0.96)	0.443[a]

Abbreviation: *NA = not applicable.*

Logistic Regression Analysis for the Effect of Independent Variables

Univariate regression analysis was used to exclude non-statistically significant variables, including coffee consumption and cerebral infarction ($P > 0.05$). The variables selected for the regression model were age, height, weight, BMI, menarche age, menopausal age, drinking tea, drinking milk, hypertension, and coronary heart disease. Multivariate regression analysis showed that hypertension was a significant influencing factor for osteoporosis ($P < 0.05$). In addition, increased age, menarche age, and milk consumption were related to an increased risk of osteoporosis. Moreover, lower height, lighter weight, and earlier menopause may also be related to the increased risk of osteoporosis (Table 8.3).

Table 8.3　Multivariate logistic regression analysis for the effect of independent variables

Factors	Univariate Logistic regression			Multivariate Logistic regression		
	OR	95% CI	*P*	OR	95% CI	*P*
Age (year)	1.061	1.046–1.076	< 0.001	1.047	1.031–1.063	< 0.001
Height (m)	0.003	0.001–0.020	< 0.001	0.053	0.007–0.421	0.006
Weight (kg)	0.971	0.960–0.982	< 0.001	0.979	0.967–0.992	0.002
BMI (kg/m^2)	0.966	0.937–0.996	0.024			
Menarche age (year)	1.063	1.015–1.113	0.009	1.061	1.012–1.114	0.015
Menopause age (year)	0.970	0.944–0.998	0.033	0.960	0.933–0.988	0.006
Drinking coffee	1.303	0.737–2.304	0.363			
Drinking tea	1.401	1.036–1.894	0.028			
Drinking milk	1.588	1.592–2.353	< 0.001	1.832	1.495–2.246	< 0.001
Hypertension	1.558	1.258–2.006	< 0.001	1.303	1.012–1.677	0.040
Coronary heart disease	1.927	1.297–2.864	0.001			
Cerebral infarction	1.395	0.593–3.280	0.445			

Abbreviations: *OR = odds ratio, CI = confidence interval.*

结　果

骨质疏松症组和非骨质疏松症组受试者特征

在排除 834 名不符合标准的参与者后，2 039 名受试者被纳入研究。这 834 人中，64 人未绝经，393 人人工绝经，其余患有其他影响骨代谢的疾病。骨质疏松症组有 678 名受试者，非骨质疏松症组有 1 361 名受试者。骨质疏松症组年龄在 47～90 岁，非骨质疏松症组年龄在 45～85 岁。统计上，患有骨质疏松症的受试者的年龄和初潮年龄明显大于未患骨质疏松症的受试者，绝经年龄更早。他们的身高也更低，体重更轻（$P < 0.001$）。此外，骨质疏松症组的骨密度明显低于非骨质疏松症组（$P < 0.001$）（表 8.1）。

表 8.1 骨质疏松症组与非骨质疏松症组受试者特征（平均值 ± 标准偏差）

因 素	总 计 （**n** = 2 039）	骨质疏松症 （**n** = 678）	非骨质疏松症 （**n** = 1 361）	**P**
年龄（岁）	62.56 ± 6.67	64.29 ± 6.71	61.70 ± 6.49	< 0.001[a]
身高（米）	1.59 ± 0.05	1.55 ± 0.05	1.56 ± 0.05	< 0.001[a]
重量（千克）	57.43 ± 8.39	56.10 ± 8.10	58.08 ± 8.46	< 0.001[a]
BMI（千克 / 平方米）	23.63 ± 3.10	23.41 ± 3.06	23.74 ± 3.12	0.023[a]
初潮年龄（岁）	15.39 ± 2.00	15.56 ± 2.10	15.31 ± 1.95	0.021[a]
绝经年龄（岁）	50.33 ± 3.33	50.10 ± 3.40	50.44 ± 3.29	0.036[a]
腰椎 BMD（克 / 立方厘米）	0.77 ± 0.15	0.65 ± 0.08	0.83 ± 0.13	< 0.001[a]
股骨颈 BMD（克 / 立方厘米）	0.73 ± 0.14	0.66 ± 0.14	0.77 ± 0.12	< 0.001[a]

缩略词：*BMI = body mass index*，*BMD = bone mineral density*，*SD = standard deviation*。

骨质疏松症组与非骨质疏松症组影响因素比较

比较两组影响因素可知，骨质疏松组患者高血压、冠心病患病率较高（$P < 0.05$）。此外，骨质疏松症组喝茶和喝牛奶的比例相对较高（$P < 0.05$）（表 8.2）。

表 8.2 骨质疏松症组与非骨质疏松症组影响因素比较（%）

因 素	总 计	骨质疏松症	非骨质疏松症	**P**
氮（%）	2 039 (100)	678 (33.25)	1 361 (66.75)	NA
喝咖啡，*n*（%）	51 (2.50)	20 (2.95)	31 (2.28)	0.360[a]
喝茶，*n*（%）	196 (9.61)	79 (11.65)	117 (8.60)	0.027[a]
饮用牛奶，*n*（%）	633 (31.04)	276 (40.71)	357 (26.23)	< 0.001[a]
高血压，*n*（%）	359 (17.61)	151 (22.27)	208 (15.28)	< 0.001[a]
冠心病，*n*（%）	104 (5.10)	50 (7.37)	54 (3.97)	0.001[a]
脑梗死，*n*（%）	22 (1.08)	9 (1.33)	13 (0.96)	0.443[a]

缩略词：*NA = not applicable*。

自变量影响的逻辑回归分析

采用单变量逻辑回归分析排除无统计学意义的变量，包括咖啡摄入量和脑梗死（$P > 0.05$）。为回归模型选择的变量是年龄、身高、体重、身体质量指数、初潮年龄、绝经年龄、喝茶、喝牛奶、高血压和冠心病。多元逻辑回归分析显示，高血压是骨质疏松症的显著影响因素（$P < 0.05$）。此外，年龄增加、初潮年龄和牛奶摄入量与骨质疏松症风险增加有关。此外，较低的身高、较轻的体重和更早的绝经也可能与骨质疏松症的风险增加有关（表 8.3）。

表 8.3　自变量影响的多元逻辑回归分析

因　素	单变量逻辑回归			多元逻辑回归		
	OR	95% CI	*P*	OR	95% CI	*P*
年龄（岁）	1.061	1.046–1.076	< 0.001	1.047	1.031–1.063	< 0.001
高度（米）	0.003	0.001–0.020	< 0.001	0.053	0.007–0.421	0.006
重量（千克）	0.971	0.960–0.982	< 0.001	0.979	0.967–0.992	0.002
BMI（千克 / 平方米）	0.966	0.937–0.996	0.024			
初潮年龄（岁）	1.063	1.015–1.113	0.009	1.061	1.012–1.114	0.015
绝经年龄（岁）	0.970	0.944–0.998	0.033	0.960	0.933–0.988	0.006
喝咖啡	1.303	0.737–2.304	0.363			
喝茶	1.401	1.036–1.894	0.028			
喝牛奶	1.588	1.592–2.353	< 0.001	1.832	1.495–2.246	< 0.001
高血压	1.558	1.258–2.006	< 0.001	1.303	1.012–1.677	0.040
冠状动脉心脏疾病	1.927	1.297–2.864	0.001			
脑梗死	1.395	0.593–3.280	0.445			

缩略词：*OR = odds ratio*，*CI = confidence interval*。

8.3.2 常用表达

1）结果表明

（1）The results/findings showed/suggested/indicated/demonstrated/revealed/documented that...

结果 / 发现显示 / 暗示 / 表明 / 证明 / 揭示 / 证明……

（2）It was found that...

发现……

（3）We found that...

我们发现……

（4）... was/were found to...

发现……

2）表示与……有关

（1）... was strongly associated with...

……与……密切相关。

（2）... was inversely correlated with...

……与……负相关。

（3）... was inversely/indirectly proportional to...

……与……成反比 / 间接成正比。

（4）... was in direct proportion to...

……与……成正比。

（5）... was compared to/with... / ... as compared with/to...

……与……相比。

3）数值表达

... was increased/decreased by/to...

……增加 / 减少了 / 到……

- 多数值表达，常采用逗号、分号或括号隔开。
- 表示数量的一部分，常用 of、out of、among 等介词。
- 用数字形式及符号来表达数值，如“+”“−”“×”“÷”“=”“≤”“≥”等。
- 表示数字对比，常用“ratio”“:”“/”“versus/v.s./v.”“rate”等。
- 表示数值范围，常用 (range) from... to...、between... and...、vary from... to...、with a range... to... 等。

4）表达统计学意义

（1）There is/was significant difference in... / between... and...

在……方面 / 之间有显著差异。

（2）The difference in... / between... and... is/was significant.

……的差异 / 之间的差异是显著的。

（3）... is/was significantly different from...

……与……有显著差异。

（4）No significant difference was found/noted/observed in... / between... and...

在……中 / 之间没有发现显著差异。

8.4 讨论（Discussion）

8.4.1 讨论部分的内容与写法

讨论亦称结论（Conclusions）或评论（Comments），是作者对研究或实验结果的综合分析和理论说明，是论文中最难写的部分。与论文的方法和结果部分相比，讨论部分的写法变化最大。其内容大致包括以下三个方面：①根据研究实验结果，正确解释产生的原因，围绕引言所提出的研究目的，说明是否能论证所提出的假说；②与国内外同类研究相比，突出本研究创新之处，提出作者的观点和见解，运用归纳、分析、推理、比较等方法，对所涉及的问题进行探讨，说明本研究的理论和实践意义；③实事求是地对本研究工作的缺陷或局限性做出评价，并说明有待解决的问题，提出今后的研究方向。

讨论部分一般由引文、讨论和结论三部分组成。作者通常用一两句话作为讨论的开场白，简要说明研究背景（有的作者会删掉引文这一部分）；引出论文所要讨论的主题，介绍总的发现及具体要点；然后将自己完成的实验结果与他人或以前的研究结果进行比较，指出不同之处并以归纳、推理、比较、演绎等方法分析其不同的可能原因，阐明本研究的理论和可能的临床意义或使用价值，最终得出结论和提出建议。

讨论部分一般不使用图表，也不整段引用文献资料，而只是摘录其观点或结论，用阿拉伯数字标出参考文献。讨论中，作者应以自己的材料为主，不宜过多地旁征博引、主次颠倒或把讨论部分写成文献综述。若对自己研究的结果轻描淡写，不做深入的分析和说明，这部分就失去了讨论意义。

【例】

With the prolongation of life expectancy, the incidence of CVD and osteoporosis is increasing. More evidence has shown common risk factors and similar pathological mechanisms between the two diseases. In this retrospective study, we found that there were 678 cases of osteoporosis among all the women who met the criteria, with a prevalence rate of 33.25%, which was similar to that reported in other studies. Among the 678 patients, 151 suffered from hypertension, and 50 suffered from coronary heart disease. The prevalence was significantly higher than that of non-osteoporosis. This illustrates that CVD may increase the risk of osteoporosis, which is consistent with previous studies. To further investigate the factors causing this increased risk, we conducted a multivariate regression analysis and found that hypertension was related to an increased risk of osteoporosis. This indicated a significant association between hypertension and osteoporosis, suggesting that fracture and CVD prevention should be considered when treating osteoporosis. According to the results, drinking milk also increased the risk of osteoporosis, which was inconsistent with previous studies. This may be related to our failure to record the duration and quantity of milk.

Some studies have reported that low BMD is superior to traditional factors, such as hyperlipidemia and smoking, in predicting the development of cardiovascular events. The lower BMD and increased bone loss rates were also associated with an increased risk of CVD in the Chinese cohort. Interestingly, a study showed a favorable relationship between a reduced risk of cardiovascular disease and BMD. Another study followed 6,872 men and women for 5.7 years, and 196 developed myocardial infarction during this period. The results revealed that low hip BMD was an influencing factor for infarction. These studies showed the relationship between low BMD and CVD.

Low BMD is a significant phenotype of osteoporosis, illustrating the relationship between osteoporosis and CVD. Osteoporosis and CVD are common age-related diseases. As shown in the results, the risk of osteoporosis increased with age. Changes in oestrogen levels caused by menopause or ageing can directly affect blood vessel walls and bone metabolism. Bones and blood vessels are considered to be important targets for oestrogen, which can improve the function of endothelial cells and vascular smooth muscle cells, inhibit platelet aggregation, and affect blood vessel responses to injury. Similarly, oestrogen in serum can reduce the number and activity of osteoclasts and inhibit bone resorption. The decrease in oestrogen results in increased bone resorption. In addition, the reduction may lead to an increase in proinflammatory cytokines, which are related to bone loss and severe arteriosclerosis.

Disorders of lipid metabolism in postmenopausal women are closely related to bone dysfunction. Dyslipidemia is also one of the pathogenic factors of hypertension, which may explain the relationship between osteoporosis and hypertension. Our results also showed that hypertension is a significant influencing factor for osteoporosis. Many clinical studies support the effect of lipid metabolism on osteoporosis. A survey of Chinese people showed that elevated levels of serum high-density lipoprotein cholesterol (HDL-C) led to higher risk of osteoporosis, but a higher HDL-C level was favorable for cardiovascular diseases. Another study indicated that femoral neck BMD in postmenopausal women was positively correlated with low-density lipoprotein cholesterol (LDL-C) and negatively correlated with HDL-C. Some clinical data from other populations also support this view. An animal study demonstrated that an atherogenic diet could lead to lower bone mineral content (BMC) and BMD. Some cytokines secreted by adipose tissue have also been shown to be involved in the regulation of bone metabolism, such as leptin and adiponectin. All these studies illustrate the correlation between lipid and bone metabolism.

A limitation of this study is that it was a single-center retrospective study with poor homogeneity, many confounding factors, and low evidence. Second, it was difficult to obtain a causal relationship between influencing factors and osteoporosis; thus, a prospective cohort study should be considered in the future. Third, the information related to cardiovascular disease came from medical records rather than immediate examination. Although we tried our best to obtain objective data, there were still some biases in personal lifestyle data. Further research needs to be performed based on this study.

Conclusion

In short, this observational study indicated an association between osteoporosis and CVD in Chinese postmenopausal women. Based on the results, cardiovascular assessment should be considered in patients with osteoporosis to prevent adverse events. This further supports the view that there is a biological link between the two.

随着预期寿命的延长，心血管疾病和骨质疏松症的发病率越来越高。更多证据表明，这两种疾病之间存在共同的危险因素和相似的病理机制。在本次回顾性研究中，我们发现符合标准的女性中有 678 例患有骨质疏松症，患病率为 33.25%，与其他研究报道的结果相似。678 例患者中，高血压 151 例，冠心病 50 例。患病率明显高于非骨质疏松症患者。这说明心血管疾病可能会增加骨质疏松症的风险，这与之前的研究一致。为了进一步调查导致这种风险增加的因素，我们进行了多元回归分析，发现高血压与骨质疏松症风险增加有关。这表明高血压与骨质疏松症之间存在显著关联，也表明在治疗骨质疏松症时应考虑预防骨折和心血管疾病。结果显示，喝牛奶还会增加患骨质疏松症的风险，这与之前的研究不一致。这可能与我们没有记录喝牛奶的时长和数量有关。

一些研究报道，低骨密度在预测心血管事件发展方面优于传统因素，如高脂血症和吸烟。在中国队列中，较低的骨密度和增加的骨丢失率也与心血管疾病风险增加有关。有趣的是，一项研究表明心血管疾病风险降低与骨密度之间存在良好关系。另一项研究对 6 872 名男性和女性进行了为期 5.7 年的随访，其中 196 人在此期间发生了心肌梗死。结果显示，低髋部骨密度是梗死的影响因素。这些研究显示了低骨密度与心血管疾病之间的关系。

低骨密度是骨质疏松症的一个重要表型，说明了骨质疏松症与心血管疾病之间的关系。骨质疏松症和心血管疾病是常见的与年龄相关的疾病。如结果所示，骨质疏松症的风险随着年龄的增长而增加。更年期或衰老引起的雌激素水平变化可直接影响血管壁和骨代谢。骨骼和血管被认为是雌激素的重要作用靶点，雌激素可以改善内皮细胞和血管平滑肌细胞的功能，抑制血小板聚集，影响血管对损伤的反应。同样，血清中的雌激素可以减少破骨细胞的数量和活性，抑制骨吸收。雌激素的减少导致骨吸收增加。此外，这种减少可能导致促炎细胞因子增加，这与骨质流失和严重动脉硬化有关。

绝经后女性脂质代谢紊乱与骨功能障碍密切相关。血脂异常也是高血压的致病因素之一，这或许可以解释骨质疏松症与高血压的关系。我们的研究结果还表明，高血压是骨质疏松症的重要影响因素。许多临床研究支持脂质代谢对骨质疏松症的影响。一项针对中国人的调查表明，血清高密度脂蛋白胆固醇水平升高会导致骨质疏松症的风险增加，但较高的高密度脂蛋白胆固醇水平有利于心血管疾病。另一项研究表明，绝经后女性的股骨颈骨密度与低密度脂蛋白胆固醇呈正相关，与高密度脂蛋白胆固醇呈负相关。来自其他人群的一些临床数据也支持这一观点。一项动物研究表明，致动脉粥样化饮食可导致较低的骨矿物质含量和骨密度。脂肪组织分泌的一些细胞因子也被证明参与了骨代谢的调节，如瘦素和脂联素。这些研究都说明了脂质和骨代谢之间的相关性。

本研究的局限性在于它是一项单中心回顾性研究，同质性差，混杂因素多，证据不足。二是难以获得影响因素与骨质疏松症的因果关系，因此未来应考虑进行前瞻性队列研究。第三，与心血管疾病相关的信息来自病历而不是即时检查。虽然我们尽力获取客观数据，但个人生活方式数据仍然存在一些偏差，需要在本研究的基础上进行进一步的研究。

结论

简而言之，这项观察性研究表明，中国绝经后女性的骨质疏松症与心血管疾病之间存在关联。基于上述结果，应考虑对骨质疏松症患者进行心血管评估，以预防不良事件发生。这进一步支持了二者之间存在生物学联系的观点。

8.4.2 常用表达

1）表示研究或结果表明的内容

（1）In this study, we provided evidence that...

在这项研究中，我们提供的证据表明……

（2）In this study, we have found that...

在这项研究中，我们发现……

（3）The evidence is that...

证据是……

（4）This study shows that...

这项研究表明……

（5）Our result indicates that...

我们的结果表明……

（6）The results are consistent with the theory that...

结果与理论一致，即……

（7）It is of great significance in...

它在……方面具有重要意义。

2）表示局限性和未来的研究方向

（1）In our experiment, we fail to show...

在我们的实验中，我们未能证明……

（2）The evidence is not likely to...

证据不太可能……

（3）The result of the test didn't support that...

测试的结果并不支持……

（4）... remains / is yet to be determined.

……还有待确定。

（5）Further analysis/experiments will be necessary/needed to confirm...

需要进一步的分析 / 实验来证实……

Exercises

Exercise I　Translate the following into Chinese.

1. Morbidity and mortality rates from atherosclerotic cardiovascular disease (ASCVD) continue to be extremely high in the world. Hypercholesterolemia is known to be a major ASCVD risk factor and the LDL-C lowering therapy has attracted extensive attention which has become a cornerstone of primary and secondary prevention in ASCVD. However, the substantial residual risk of ASCVD often remains after adjustment for the certain risk factors such as LDL-C or intensive LDL-C lowering with statins and other optimal therapies. The Residual Risk Reduction Initiative (R3i) has previously highlighted atherogenic dyslipidemia, defined as the imbalance between proatherogenic triglyceride-rich apolipoprotein B-containing-lipoproteins and anti-atherogenic apolipoprotein A1-lipoproteins (as in high density lipoprotein, HDL), as an important modifiable contributor to lipid-related residual cardiovascular risk. Recently, pieces of evidence

are accumulating to suggest that hypertriglyceridemia is causally associated with increased atherosclerosis risk. This article will review relevant literature regarding the association between hypertriglyceridemia and atherosclerosis including clinical studies and the researches of proatherogenic mechanism.

2. Obesity is both a major risk factor and a disease modifier of asthma in children and adults. While obesity is defined according to a threshold BMI, recent studies suggest that BMI z-scores may be unreliable, particularly among children and adolescents with severe obesity. In adults, obesity is defined as a BMI of 30 kg/m^2 or more, yet a given BMI may reflect vastly differing physiology and metabolic health. This distinction is likely important for asthma: while serum interleukin-6 (IL-6) (produced by macrophages in adipose tissue, and a marker of metabolic health) is a marker of asthma severity, some individuals with BMI's in the non-obese range have elevated IL-6; Sideleva et al. found that adipose tissue inflammation is increased in obese individuals with asthma, compared with obese controls. Metabolic dysfunction is more important than fat mass for asthma in obesity. However, most asthma studies have used BMI and metabolic dysfunction related to obesity synonymously; in this article, we will report data on metabolic dysfunction where available, but will otherwise use obesity as a marker of both fat mass and metabolic dysfunction.

Exercise II　List appropriate subheadings for each subsection in this "Methods" section. Put the list in optimal order.

Subheadings:

Study Design

Participants

Methods of Measurement

Statistical Analysis

1. Newly diagnosed women with GDM between 24–28 weeks-of-gestation who attended the Antenatal Care Clinic and met the inclusion criteria were invited to participate in the study. GDM was diagnosed based on the International Association of Diabetes and Pregnancy Study Groups criteria as follows: fasting plasma glucose ⩾ 92 mg/dL at the first prenatal visit, or an abnormal glucose tolerance test at 24–28 weeks-of-gestation using a 75g oral glucose load (defined as one or more of the following abnormal glucose values: fasting plasma glucose ⩾ 92 mg/dL, 1–h ⩾ 180 mg/dL, 2–h ⩾ 153 mg/dL). Other inclusion criteria included: ① singleton pregnancy; ② maternal age of 18–45 years old; ③ normal fetal structures or chromosomes based on ultrasound scanning during the second trimester and/or invasive prenatal diagnosis; and ④ no history of chronic diseases, such as immunodeficiency, hypertension, pre-gestational

diabetes, kidney disease, or liver disease. Exclusion criteria included: ① consuming probiotic food products, such as yogurt, fermented foods and bean paste during the 2 weeks before enrollment; and ② exposure to antibiotics during the 4 weeks before enrollment.

2. Data were analyzed using the SPSS statistical software package version 22 IBM (International Business Machines Corp.), Armonk, New York, the U.S. The variables were expressed as means (standard deviation) and *n* (%). After testing data for normality, two-sample t-tests or Mann-Whitney tests were used to compare continuous variables between the two groups at the baseline as appropriate. The χ2-test and Fisher's exact tests were used to compare categorical data. Mean differences in the changes in metabolic parameters during the intervention period between the two groups were compared by independent t-tests. *P*-values < 0.05 were considered statistically significant.

3. A double-blind, placebo-controlled, randomized clinical trial was carried out between June 2016 and February 2017 at the Antenatal Care Clinic, Faculty of Medicine, Ramathibodi Hospital, Mahidol University, Bangkok, Thailand. This study was reviewed and approved by the Committee on Human Rights Related to Research Involving Human Subjects, Faculty of Medicine, Ramathibodi Hospital, and complied with the Declaration of Helsinki. Written informed consent was obtained from all participants. The study was registered at the Thai clinical trials registry, number 20170606002.

4. All participants were randomly allocated to take one capsule containing either a probiotic or placebo once daily after the morning meal for four consecutive weeks. The probiotic used in this study was Infloran® (Laboratorio Farmaceutico SIT, Mede, Italy, and imported by DKSH, Bangkok, Thailand). It is commercially available at Ramathibodi Hospital, where it has been used for the treatment of acute non-specific enterocolitis and chronic constipation. Each capsule contained 1,000 million CFU of Lactobacillus acidophilus and 1,000 million CFU of Bifidobacterium bifidum. This dose was similar to that utilized in previous studies 18, 20. Each placebo capsule contained gelatin. Participants were counseled to avoid probiotic-containing foods and supplements throughout the study period to minimize the confounding from other probiotics. Participants were given a 2-week package of either probiotic or placebo capsules and instructed to refrigerate them at 4 ℃. They were seen every 2 weeks at our antenatal care clinic for standard antenatal treatment, monitoring compliance with the treatment and monitoring for adverse effects from the interventions. Compliance monitoring was carried out by capsule count. Afterwards, a second 2-week package of either probiotic or placebo capsules was given to the patients. Additionally, weekly telephone follow-up calls were carried out to encourage compliance with the assigned intervention and to monitor for any possible adverse events.

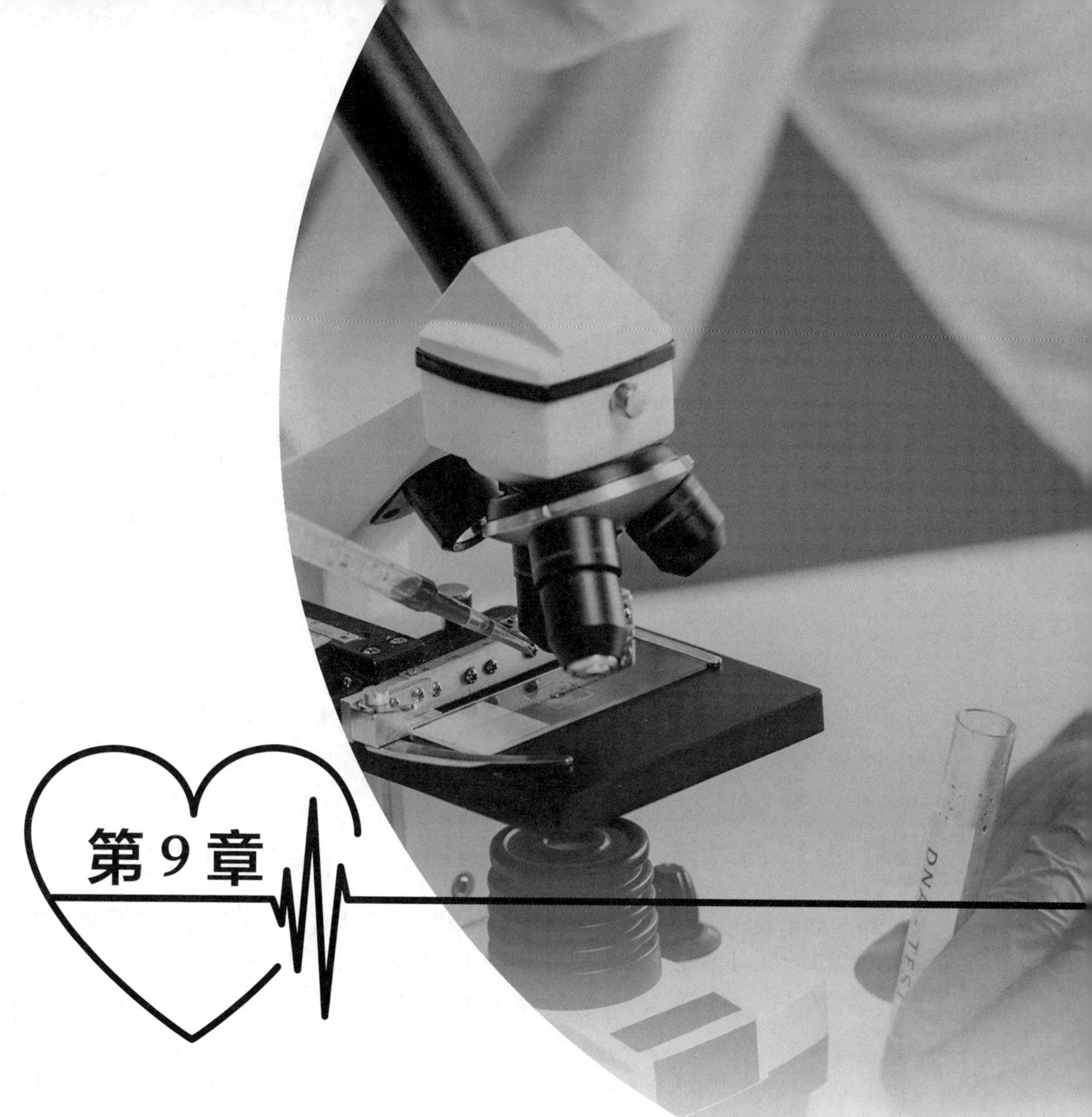

第 9 章

医学研究论文 II（Medical Research Papers II）

A picture is worth a thousand words.

一图胜千言。

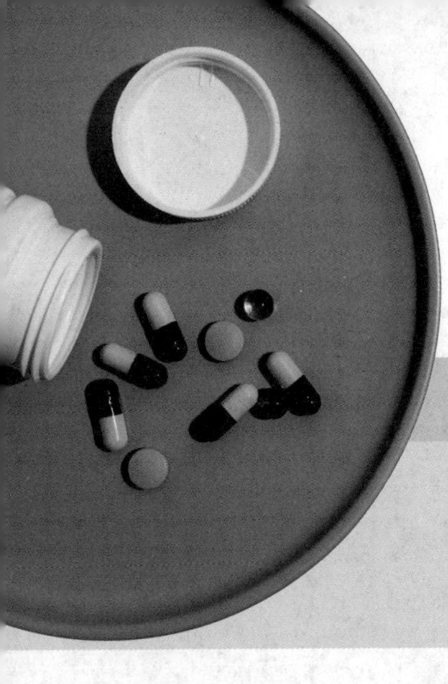

Warm-up

1. How to justify your point of view by the use of data?
2. Please list some common forms of graph.

上一章介绍了医学论文的主体部分，本章将介绍论文中出现的表格、插图、致谢、参考文献及医学伦理等内容。

9.1 表格与插图（Tables and Illustrations）

表格与插图是医学类英语论文写作的重要表述方式之一。有些医学内容过于繁杂，难以用文字表述清楚，而表图可以起到画龙点睛的作用，能够形象地表述技术手段、实验结果、科学思想等内容，使读者较为直观地了解研究成果，获取相关信息。

在《生物医学期刊投稿的统一要求》中，投稿论文的表格需排在参考文献的后面，每个表格占一页。图注另起一页，排在表格的后面。插图放在图注之后，也是每个图占一页。

9.1.1 表图的结构（Structure of Tables and Illustrations）

表格一般为三线表，包括表号（Table No.）、表题（Titles）、栏目（Headings）、线条（Lines）、数字（Figures）和表注（Footnotes）等。

插图一般分为线条图和照片图。线条图反映变量之间的定量关系，而照片图能真实且直观地传递信息。常用的线条图有统计图和示意图。统计图主要包括图题（Titles）、标目（Headings）、比例（Scales）、图线（Lines）、图例（Legends）和图注（Footnotes）等。照片图应做到清晰度高、对比度好。

【例】

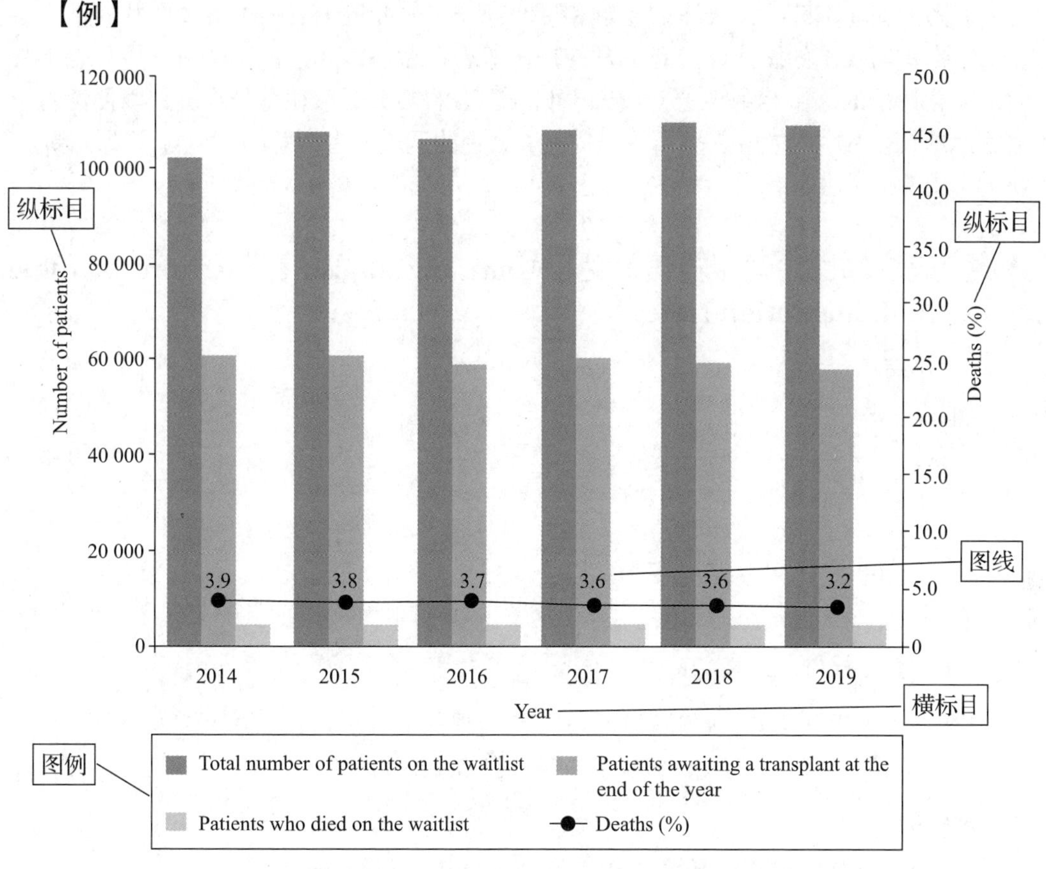

Figure 9.1 Number of waitlisted patients and patients dying on the waiting list in the EU from 2014 to 2019.

The percentage of deaths is calculated as the ratio of those who died that year while waitlisted to the total number active on the waiting list that year multiplied by 100. There was a 7% increase in the number waitlisted over this 5-year period. The percentage of deaths remained relatively stable between 3%–4%. Data were calculated based on data from the Transplant Newsletter135.

9.1.2 表图的英文表达规范（English Expression Norms of Tables and Illustrations）

表图标题应做到简明扼要，概括表图的主题，突出要点。

一般来说，表图标题第一个单词的首字母要大写，某些虚词（如介词、冠词、连词等）要小写，不定式中的 to 要小写。标题中实词（如名词、代词、形容词、副词、动词等）的首字母要大写，同时涵盖连字符连接单词的第二部分首字母，如 Blood-Based。一些医学类英语期刊对表图的标题要求没有那么严格，只需将第一个单词的首字母和专有名词大写即可。

表图的图注部分，即表图的注解和说明部分，一般位于表的上方和图片的下方或旁边。在撰写表图的图注时，我们常使用一般现在时态，如描述某个科学原理、不受时间变化影响的某个客观现象，或者说明表图中的某个图形和符号含义，以便读者更清晰地理解表图中的内容。然而，当描述表图中的调查或者实验的研究方法或结果时，我们常用一般过去时态。

9.1.3 表注和图注常用英语表达（Common English Expressions of Table and Illustration Notes）

1）总结

summary of...

总结……

2）影响

effect/influence of... on... in...

在……中……对……的影响

3）观察（报告、结果）

an observation / observations of/on/in... and... / ... with... / between... and...

对……和……/……与……/……和……之间的观察

4）调查

survey/investigation of/on... and... / of... with... / between... and...

对……和……/……与……/……和……之间的调查

5）关系 / 相关 / 比较 / 对照

relationship/correlation/association/comparison/contrast of... and... / of... with... / between... and...

……和……/……与……/……和……之间的关系 / 关联 / 比较 / 对比

6）资料来源

Data are adapted/taken from...

数据改编 / 取自……

9.1.4 示例（Examples of Table and Illustration Notes）

【例 1】

Figure 1 Summary of results of dietary programs network meta-analysis at last follow-up

图 1 饮食计划网络荟萃分析最后随访结果总结

【例 2】

Table 2 Display of the 30-day and 1-year mortality rates for both control group and experimental group

表 2 显示了对照组和实验组的 30 天和 1 年的死亡率

【例 3】

CI indicates confidence interval

CI 表示置信区间

【例 4】

Figure 2 Example of How HealthMap Uses Natural-Language Processing to Classify Infectious-Disease Case Reports

图 2 健康地图如何使用自然语言处理对传染病病例报告进行分类的示例

【例 5】

Table 1 New SARS-CoV-2 Infections Among Vaccinated Health Care Workers from December 16, 2020, through February 9, 2021

表 1 2020 年 12 月 16 日至 2021 年 2 月 9 日接种疫苗的医护人员中新感染的严重急性呼吸系统综合征冠状病毒 2 型

9.2 致谢（Acknowledgements）

致谢是论文作者对推动本研究进展、协助论文完成和发表、对论文有一定的贡献但又并非作者的相关组织或个人的感谢，主要感谢为论文提供帮助、指导、审核的相关人员和在研究中提供技术、资金、设备的相关单位、机构组织、人员以及可能发生利益冲突的相关者。根据医学期刊要求，致谢内容须征得被致谢人、被致谢单位和组织的同意。

9.2.1 致谢位置（The Position of Acknowledgements）

致谢的内容常置于论文正文后、参考文献前，用英文 Acknowledgements 表示；致谢内容也可放在论文首页的脚注中，如基金资助项目常以脚注的形式出现在论文首页。致谢部分并不属于论文正文，英文字体比正文小一号。

注意：并非所有的论文都有致谢内容。

9.2.2 常用英语表达（Common English Expressions of Acknowledgements）

1）基金资助来源：表明研究得到某单位、某组织、某人的支持和资助

（1）本课题为国家自然科学基金资助项目 + 项目资助号，如：

The research was supported by the National Natural Science Foundation of China (No. XXXXXX).

本研究得到了国家自然科学基金的资助（项目编号：XXXXXX）。

（2）本课题为国家杰出青年科学基金资助的课题 + 项目资助号，如：

The project was supported by the National Science Foundation for Distinguished Young Scholars of China (No. XXXXXX).

本项目得到了国家杰出青年科学基金的资助（项目编号：XXXXXX）。

（3）本课题为某省自然科学基金资助项目 + 项目资助号，如：

The research was supported by the Natural Science Foundation of XXX Province of China (No. XXXXXX).

本研究得到了中国 XXX 省自然科学基金的资助（项目编号：XXXXXX）。

（4）本研究得到了世界卫生组织的资助，如：

The research was supported by the World Health Organization.

本研究得到了世界卫生组织的支持。

（5）对本研究做出贡献的其他研究人员，如：

Other investigators who contributed to this study were...

其他参与这项研究的研究者是……

2）致谢表达方式：表示对某单位、某组织及某人的感谢

（1）thank... for...，如：

We thank Chinese Preventive Medicine Association for providing financial support.

我们感谢中华预防医学会提供的资助。

（2）express... thanks to... for...，如：

The authors would like to express thanks to Professor Liu for reviewing the manuscript.

作者感谢刘教授审读了手稿。

（3）be thankful to... for...，如：

The authors are thankful to Professor Wang for technical assistance.

作者感谢王教授给予技术帮助。

（4）be grateful to... for...，如：

The authors are grateful to Dr. Zhang for clinical help.

作者感谢张博士给予的临床帮助。

（5）be appreciated...，如：

The statistical analysis of this study by Professor Wang is appreciated by the authors.

作者感谢王教授给予本研究的统计学分析。

9.3 参考文献（References）

参考文献是医学科研论文的重要组成部分，既反映了作者对他人学术成果的尊重，表明论文依据的科学性，又便于读者查阅相关资料。二十大报告提出，要在全社会“弘扬诚信文化，健全诚信建设长效机制”。在科研论文中，标明他人作品及科研数据出处，尊重和保护他人的著作权，弘扬实事求是、严谨执着的科研精神，是每一个科研工作者的责任与义务。

9.3.1 参考文献的要求（The Requirements of References）

1）选用原则：准确性、关联性、时效性

作者必须阅读引用的文献且保证出处准确，确保读者能根据文献信息查找到对应的文献；注重选择最主要且与论文内容有密切关联的文献，最好是行业领域内的专家文献，提高信服度。此外，文献要有时效性，最好是近 3～5 年公开发表过的文献。

2）引用数量

国内医学期刊的论文引用文献一般在 10 条左右，国外医学期刊的论文引用文献的数量不一，少则 10 多条，多则 200 条以上。

3）位置安排

参考文献是论文的最后一部分，国内医学期刊一般要求中文文献在前、英文文献在后，通常用阿拉伯数字进行顺序排列。

9.3.2 参考文献的格式（The Format of References）

医学英语论文的参考文献格式广泛遵循《生物医学期刊投稿的统一要求》，被简称为温哥华格式。国际医学期刊编辑委员会于 1978 年首次发表温哥华格式，之后进行多次修改。国际医学期刊编辑委员会包含《内科学年鉴》《柳叶刀》（*The Lancet*）、《美国医学会杂志》（*The Journal of the American Medical Association*，*JAMA*）等 16 个正式成员期刊和组织，在国际医学期刊领域拥有广泛的影响力。国内多数医学期刊也按照温哥华格式编排稿件。温哥华格式对参考文献的具体要求如下：

（1）参考文献按照其在正文中出现的先后顺序排列，用阿拉伯数字连续编写，在正文引文句末的右上角位置标明数字；若一篇文章被多次引用，仍使用同一编号，以首次引用的序号为准；若出现两篇相连的序号，则用逗号分开，如[1, 2]；若出现三篇及以上相连的序号，则用起止号，如 [1-3]；有的医学期刊则用方括号表示，如 [1, 2]、[1-3]。例如：

Patients with coronary artery disease (CAD) are considered to be at high risk or very high risk for future adverse cardiovascular events.[1, 2]

（2）参考文献标题通常用 References（首字母大写）或 REFERENCES（全部字母大写）来表示。

（3）标准期刊参考文献格式为：作者. 题名. 期刊名称. 年份；卷（期）：起止页。例如：

Mink S, Schwarz U, Mudra R, Gugl C, Fröhlich J, Keller E. Treatment of resistant fever: new method of local cerebral cooling. *Neurocrit Care*. 2011; 15(1): 107–112.

（4）温哥华格式要求列出六位以内的作者，人名用逗号隔开，最后用点号结束；如果作者超过六位，列出前六位作者，后加 et al.；应将作者的姓放置第一位，且首字母大写，作者的名则缩写，置于姓后，如 William Ramsay 应写为 Ramsay W。如果作者有两个名，则将两个名的缩写连在一起，如 Linus Carl Pauling 应写为 Pauling LC，William Howard Stein 应写为 Stein WH。例如：

Guilbert TW, Morgan WJ, Zeiger RS, Mauger DT, Boehmer SJ, Szefler SJ, et al. Long-term inhaled corticosteroids in preschool children at high risk for asthma. *NEJM*. 2006; 354(19): 1985–1997.

9.4 医学伦理（Medical Ethics）

本教材深入贯彻党的二十大精神，弘扬和践行当代中国人权观，坚持“人民至上、生命至上”的理念。在医学研究中，我们要尊重、保护研究参与者的合法权益，规范医学研究伦理审查工作。

国内外权威医学期刊对伦理学的要求主要依据以下文件：①《生物医学期刊投稿的统一要求》的第二部分“生物医学研究和报道的伦理学问题”；②曾于 1975 年制定、2000 年修订的《赫尔辛基宣言》；③（所在单位和国家）人体试验委员会制定的伦理标准；④（所在单位和国家）有关实验动物管理、使用的规定等。

9.4.1 主要内容（Main Content）

1）隐私和保护

作者应注意保护患者隐私，未经患者同意，不得侵犯其隐私权。若因科研需要，作者须获得患者的知情同意，让患者过目有可能辨别其身份的材料。如果临床试验对象涉及胎儿、儿童或认知障碍弱势群体，作者必须征得父母或监护人的知情同意，才可刊登患者有关信息，如文字描述、照片等。在刊登时，作者应遮盖可辨认患者身份的细节。一般情况下，期刊会要求作者出具患者的知情同意书，并在致谢部分说明情况。

2）受试人与动物的保护

遵循《赫尔辛基宣言》的同时，以人为研究对象的试验报告，作者在研究方法部分还应说明是否经过相关伦理委员会的审查批准、是否经过受试对象知情同意。若有期刊要求提供伦理委员会的批准文件、患者知情同意书，作者应按照其要求，提前设计研究。以动物为研究对象的实验，作者应说明其是否遵循其国家、研究机构制定的有关实验动物管理及使用的规定。

3）作者与贡献者

作者的署名体现了道德规范，作者应是对发表的研究成果有实质性贡献的人，必须至少承当研究中的某部分工作，而且作者的排名顺序应按照其贡献大小排列。贡献者指的是对论文的发表有一定帮助但达不到作者资格的人，如提供技术帮助、参与研究调查、给予一般性支持的人。作者可在致谢中感谢他们，同时须注意，致谢这批人，须征得其同意。

9.4.2 常用英语表达（Common English Expressions）

一般来说，按照期刊要求，作者必须在医学论文的材料、研究方法部分用文字明确说明受试对象是否符合上文中提到的标准，常见英语表达如下所示：

1）医学研究涉及人类受试者的情况

The protocol **was approved by** the XXX Hospital Ethics Committee and the study was conducted **in accordance with** the Declaration of Helsinki. Written informed consent **was obtained from** all participants.

该协议经 XXX 医院伦理委员会批准，根据《赫尔辛基宣言》进行研究，并获得了所有受试者的知情同意书。

2）医学研究涉及受试体是动物的情况

（1）The research proposals **were approved by** XXX Committee.

本研究提案经过了 XXX 委员会批准。

（2）All animal experiments were conducted **in accordance with** principles stated in Guide for the Care and Use of Laboratory Animals.

所有动物实验均按照《实验动物的护理和使用指南》中规定的原则进行。

（3）These experiments **were approved by** the Animal Care Committee of XXX University.

这些实验得到了 XXX 大学动物护理委员会的批准。

3）医学研究中致谢部分的科研道德情况

注意：作者须清晰罗列致谢对象的具体贡献。

（1）The authors thank XXX **who participated in** the study.

作者感谢参与本研究的 XXX。

（2）We are thankful to XXX **for gathering information**.

我们非常感谢 XXX 收集的信息。

（3）The authors thank XXX, XXX, XXX, who **cared for** the study patients.

作者感谢照顾研究患者的 XXX、XXX、XXX。

（4）We wish to express our appreciation to XXX Institute **for their assistance**.

我们想要对 XXX 研究所的协助表示感谢。

Exercises

Exercise I　Translate the following into English.

1. 表 3 接受溶栓疗法或经皮腔内冠状动脉成形术（PTCA）治疗患者的住院记录
2. 图 2 每名参与者饮用咖啡后和避免咖啡因情况下的睡眠分钟数
3. 作者对欧阳先生提供图片表示真诚的感谢。
4. 我们感谢中国医学研究会提供的资助。
5. 下列动物实验方案经过了 XXX 大学实验动物伦理委员会审核。

Exercise II　Translate the following into Chinese.

1. Figure 1 Various Functions of Artificial Intelligence (AI) for Infectious-Disease Surveillance
2. Table 2 Summary of all-cause mortality results at last follow-up for named dietary programs versus minimal intervention
3. All subjects gave their informed consent for inclusion before they participated in the study. The study was conducted in accordance with the Declaration of Helsinki, and the protocol was approved by the Ethics Committee of XXX.
4. The statistical analysis of this study by Professor Alex Smith is acknowledged.
5. Shown is a non-exhaustive list of functions of AI-aided infectious disease surveillance and representative examples from the published literature.

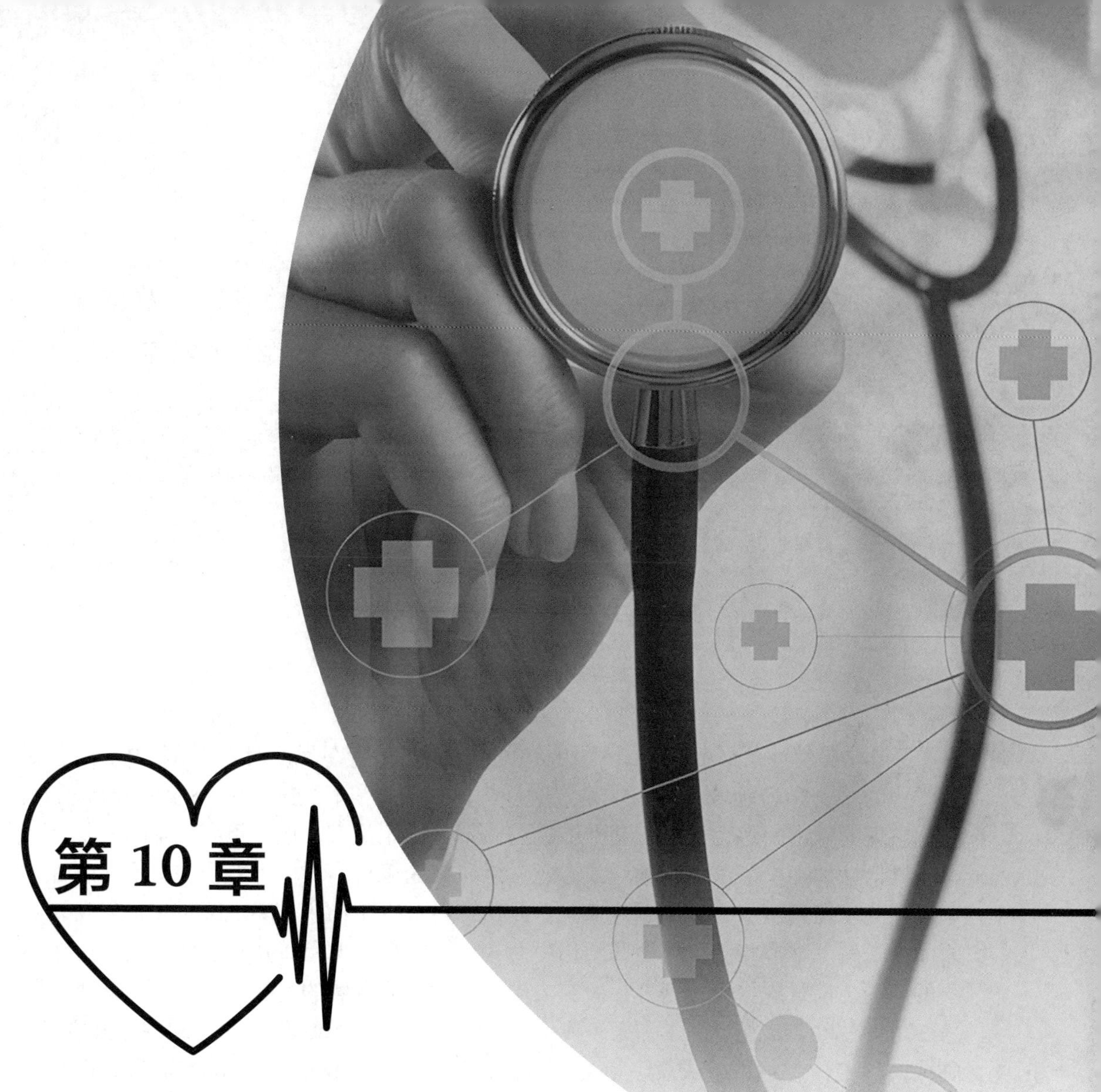

第 10 章

医学文献综述（Medical Literature Review）

By the side of sickness health becomes sweet.

生病方知健康贵。

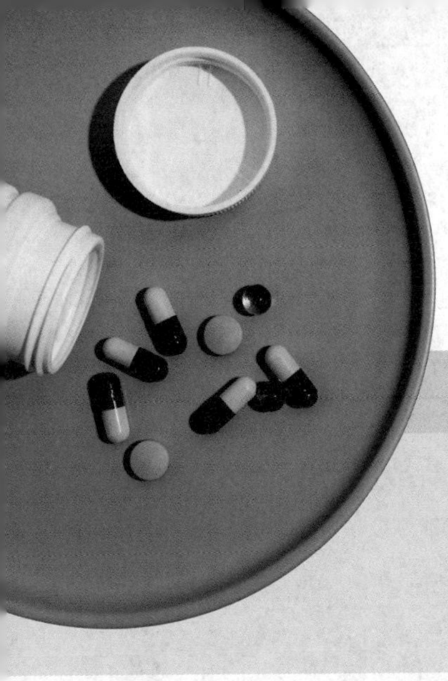

Warm-up

1. What is a literature review? Have you ever conducted a literature review?
2. What's the purpose of a literature review?

医学文献综述（Medical Literature Review）是作者在阅读相关文献的基础上，对医学中的某一学科领域或专题在特定时间内的情报资料，进行全面系统的分析研究、归纳整理而做出的综合评述。文献综述虽然不是原始论文，但一篇高质量的文献综述等于概括性地评析了该学科领域或专题学术研究的概貌。作者可能会在一篇文献综述中引用几十篇乃至上百篇原始论文。由此，综述可以帮助研究者、医学工作者在较短时间内了解、掌握相关研究课题的历史背景、研究现状、争论焦点、已解决和尚未解决的问题、前景展望等，是选择研究方向、寻找科研课题的重要线索来源。此外，随着 20 世纪 90 年代循证医学临床实践（evidence-based clinical practice）时代的到来，临床医学工作者越来越依靠医学文献综述，权衡各种疗法优劣，指导临床医疗决策。本章重点讲述医学文献综述的特点、类型、写作步骤及结构与写法。

10.1 综述的特点（Features of Literature Review）

1. 新颖性

综述不是简单记录学科发展的历史，而是要搜集最新资料，获取最新内容，将最新的医学信息和科研动向及时传递给读者。普赖斯指数（Price's Indicator）指在一个具体学科内，把对年限不超过五年的引文数量与引文总数之比作为指标，用以测量文献的老化速度与程度。普赖斯指数越高，越能反映文献综述的新颖程度，也越易于引导或发表新课题研究。

2. 综合性

综述应紧紧围绕中心论题旁征博引，做到放得开、收得拢，即为了集中于焦点，广泛综述国内外的相关研究成果。

3. 评述性

在综述文献的基础上，作者应对所引用的原理、方法、成果或结论等发表自己的意见，而非罗列堆砌文献。这一点对专业研究人员写作文献综述来说尤为重要，因为它可能决定所写文献综述是否有发表价值。

4. 准确客观性

作者应尽可能阅读原刊发表的论文或其复印件，确保读懂原意，以免断章取义或以讹传讹；既要注意引证与自己观点相同的文献，也要引证其他文献；发表观点和见解时，须做到论据充足、分析客观，决不臆断、拔高。

10.2 综述类型（Types of Literature Review）

根据综述目的、内容、研究范围和问题，综述有不同的分类。格兰特（Grant）等研究人员列举了 14 种综述类型及相关方法，对其进行了描述性的概括和举例。他们使用了与循证医学原则相一致的分析方法，即检索（search）、评估（appraisal）、综合（synthesis）、分析（analysis）来识别每种综述类型及相关方法，并对其优缺点和应用范围进行总结，帮助研究者更容易地了解和区分各种综述类型。这里主要介绍其中四种常见的文献综述类型：传统文献综述、系统综述、荟萃分析和范围综述。这四种类型的文献综述方法虽存在一定的相似之处，但其本质上还存在较大差别。传统文献综述常是硕博学位论文的一部分，也可单独成文。相较于传统文献综述，系统综述、荟萃分析和范围综述有其固定的步骤、检索的广泛性、设计的严谨性，因此其证据水平更高，更易于被国际期刊录用发表，近年来受到研究者的青睐。研究者应根据具体的研究问题和目的选择最为合适的综述方法。

10.2.1 传统文献综述（Literature Review）

传统文献综述可以指广义上的文献综述，也可指狭义上的传统文献综述。传统文献综述是指研究者根据特定目的、需要或兴趣，围绕某一主题收集相关的医学文献，采用定性分析的方法，对论文的研究目的、方法、结果、结论和观点等进行分析和评价，并结合自己的观点和临床经验进行阐述和评论，最终总结成文。传统文献综述也可进一步细分，大致可分为文摘性综述和分析性综述两种。文摘性综述又称综合文摘，是对原始文献进行客观的综合性摘述，以提供详尽的资料为目的，不掺杂撰写者本人的观点，由读者对综述的内容做出判断。分析性综述通过对原始文献的内容进行分析后表达作者的意见和见解，既有回顾，又有瞻望，可以提出问题，也可以提炼新思路、新方法。该类型一般缺乏严格的程序和步骤，缺乏标准化、可重复的方法。“护士职业倦怠及应对策略文献综述”（Burnout and coping strategies among nurses: A literature review）、“基于计算机的患者教育方法的文献综述”（Computer-based approaches to patient education: A review of the literature）、“老年患者接受联合放射治疗、免疫疗法和靶向药物的安全性和有效性的文献综述”（Safety and efficacy of combined radiotherapy, immunotherapy, and targeted agents in elderly patients: A literature review）皆属于传统文献综述类型。

10.2.2 系统综述（Systematic Review）

系统综述是指针对某一具体临床问题，系统、全面地收集所有已发表或未发表的临床研究，采用临床流行病学严格评价文献的原则和方法，筛选出符合质量标准的文献，并采用适当的统计学方法进行定性或定量的合成，从而得出可靠的结论。它采用严格、系统的方法，评价、分析和合成多个有争议甚至相互矛盾的小型临床研究，以解决纷争和提出建议。从方法学上看，它可分为随机对照试验的系统评价、非随机对照试验的系统评价、观察性研究的系统评价、诊断试验的系统评价等。进行研究设计时，系统综述有严格的纳入与排除标准，对于量化研究综述，作者一般采用 PICOS 结构框架：P 指 Population（研究对象），I 指 Intervention（干预或治疗方式），C 指 Comparison（方法比较），O 指 Outcome（结果），S 指 Study Design（研究设计）。对于质性文献研究综述，作者一般采用 SPIDER 结构框架：S 指 Sample（研究对象样本人群），PI 指 Phenomenon of Interest（有趣的研究现象），D 指 Design（研究设计），E 指 Evaluation（评估方法），R 指 Research Type（研究类型）。“痴呆症临终界定的系统综述”（Defining end of life in dementia: A systematic review）、“住院患者精神错乱症状的发生和结果的系统文献综述”（Occurrence and outcome of delirium in medical in-patients: A systematic literature review）、“妊娠创伤患者管理的系统文献综述”（Management of the pregnant trauma patient: A systematic literature review）皆属于系统综述类型。

10.2.3 荟萃分析（Meta-Analysis）

荟萃分析又称 Meta 分析，是一种统计学技术，即将多个研究结果合并成一个量化指标的一种技术。简单地说，荟萃分析就是同质的量性研究的统计学整合，通过统计学的方法，将多个主要研究的证据进行整合，从而保证了结果的客观性和有效性。荟萃分析既有完全随机设计，也有析因设计。因此，荟萃分析不等于系统综述，采用了荟萃合并的系统综述才能叫荟萃分析，否则就只能被称为系统综述。与一般的系统综述相比，荟萃分析可以对干预效果进行更加准确的估计。“地中海式饮食和健康状况关系的荟萃分析”（Adherence to Mediterranean diet and health status: Meta-analysis）、“患者依从性与治疗结果的荟萃分析”（Patient adherence and medical treatment outcomes: A meta-analysis）皆属于荟萃分析类型。

10.2.4 范围综述（Scoping Review）

范围综述是指为了快速描述一个研究领域的关键概念、主要资源和可及证据种类的研究所进行的综述。它可用于探索一类研究的范围、程度和本质，总结和推广研究结果，并指出现存研究的不足与差距，也可用来确定某一研究问题是否有价值进行系统综述，尤其适用于覆盖面较广、内容很复杂或从未被全面研究过的新问题。2005 年，希拉里 · 阿克希（Hilary Arksey）和丽莎 · 奥玛利（Lisa O'Malley）首次提出了开展范围综述的研究框架。“医学专业人员面对围产期死亡的经历及需求范围综述”（The experiences and needs of healthcare professionals facing perinatal death: A scoping review）、“对患者医疗旅游体验的范围综述”（What is known about the patient's experience of medical tourism? A scoping review）皆属于范围综述类型。

10.3 综述写作步骤（Steps of Review Writing）

综述一般取材于他人的研究成果，有针对性地大量阅读文献资料是写好综述的基本条件。此外，综述者的综合表达能力和写作技巧也是撰写综述的基本功。撰写综述绝非简单的文献“摘抄录入”，其主要程序依次为：选题→查阅资料→提纲→资料分类→组织卡片→粗、精读论文→拟写作提纲→起草→补充、删节→修改→审核→再修改→成文。

10.3.1 选题（Subjects）

能否写出高质量的综述，选题恰当与否至关重要，原则上视作者所从事专业、专长及科研工作需要而定，应避免重复他人已发表的文献综述，现可以通过提前网上注册以避免文献综述重复发表。

常见的选题范围：①所从事的专业领域、专长项目、已进行或正在开展的研究工作，具有一定的经验和资料；②对某一专题已积累了大量的文献资料，能够提出新的进展性观点；③在实践中发现了新问题，同行间尚未形成共识，需加以总结；④从事的研究领域近年来有重大突破或进展，须深入探讨或有必要介绍给读者；⑤新发现的病种，新的诊断方法、治疗手段，新药应用于临床，尚无统一的标准或结论性共识，须对其归纳整理；⑥对某种疾病诊治观点有了新认识和见解，需要推广与应用；⑦临床、科研工作中亟须解决的课题；⑧基础理论研究中的新进展、新观点；⑨各学科间的相互联系或边缘交叉学科中的新动态等。

10.3.2 文献收集（Literature Collection）

文献资料是撰写文献综述的物质基础，确定综述的选题后，作者要大量搜集和阅读相关的中外文文献。文献越多，综述的质量就越高。选择文献时，作者应先看近期（近 3～5 年）的文献，后看远期的，在广泛阅读资料的基础上，再深入复习几篇有代表性的文章，必须阅读原文，特别是应细读具有权威性的文章。阅读文献过程中，作者应做好读书卡片或笔记，为撰写综述准备资料。现在收集文献的方法通常是使用关键词，通过电子文献数据库、学术搜索引擎等方法收集，可在短时间内收集大量相关文献，然后通过筛选，特别是系统综述等方式，根据研究问题制定严格的纳入和排除标准，剔除与主题无关或不符合入选条件的文献。常用的中文数据库有中国知网、万方医学、维普数据库等，常用的英文数据库包括 PubMed、CINAHL、Embase、Web of Science、Science Direct 等。

10.3.3 拟定提纲与写作（Outline and Writing）

完成上述步骤后，作者对选题所涉及的国内外现状及存在问题已有了概括性认识，再将精心选取的文献资料按选题要求分类、归纳及整理，按照选题的中心意图，确定论文的层次和标题，草拟出综述提纲。一般来讲，在大量获取文献的过程中，作者的构思与提纲已逐渐形成，对提纲经过仔细斟酌、推敲，必要时再调整或修正后，即可开始撰写综述。在写作过程中，作者可根据需要调整结构和补充内容。完成初稿后，作者要反复修改和补充，包括内容增减、结构统一、数据核对和文字润色等。综述发表前，作者最好请有关专家和同行审阅，力求做到主题明确、层次清楚、数据可靠、文字精练、表达准确。

10.4 综述结构与写作（Review Structure and Writing）

医学综述结构一般包括题目（Title）、作者（Author）、摘要（Abstract）、关键词（Keywords）、引言（Introduction）、综述正文（Body）、结论（Conclusion）、文献（References）等部分。综述正文部分一般包括综述方法（Methods）、结果（Results）、讨论（Discussion），传统文献综述的这一部分结构较为灵活，没有严格限制。为了便于学习写作，我们将以一篇传统医学综述文章《急诊室临终关怀综述》（"A Literature Review on Care at the End-of-Life in the Emergency Department"）为例，详细剖析其结构和写作方法。该文章选自《国际急诊医学》（*Emergency Medicine International*）期刊。

10.4.1 题目（Title）

综述题目一般含有 review、literature review、systematic review、scoping review、critical review 等标志词明示综述类型，同时包含所综述内容的核心要素，如 A Literature Review on Care at the End-of-Life in the Emergency Department 包含临终关怀和急诊室两个核心要素，literature review 表明了其为传统综述类型。作者有时也用 advances、recent advances、update、progress、evolution 等词来写综述题目，如 New trends in head and neck imaging（头颈影像学新趋势）、Evolution of the concept of self-care and implications for nurses: A literature review（自我护理概念的演变及其对护士的影响：文献综述）。医学文献综述的题目不宜过大，从某一个侧面入手更容易深入研究，题目越具体越容易收集资料，一般 8～12 个单词为宜。例

如，Pancreatic disease（胰腺疾病）这个题目太大，而 Challenges in diagnosing subclinical pancreatic disease（亚临床胰腺疾病诊断面临的挑战）这个题目更精确。题目可用一般现在时，表明研究结果的普遍有效性，也可用过去式，表明研究结果尚未得到很好的证实。

10.4.2 摘要和关键词（Abstract and Keywords）

1. 内容和要求

摘要因综述类型及期刊要求不同而有不同的写法，有的摘要类型格式自由，没有固定结构，如传统文献综述。有的摘要类型或期刊要求有固定的结构式摘要，需要简明扼要地介绍研究目的、研究方法、结果、结论。摘要长度一般为 200～500 个单词。时态一般用现在时、现在完成时和过去式。关键词一般为 3～5 个，个别综述可省略关键词。

《急诊室临终关怀综述》的英文摘要如下所示：

Abstract

The hospitalization and management of patients at the end-of-life by emergency medical services are presenting a challenge to our society as the majority of people approaching death explicitly state that they want to die at home and the transition from acute care to palliation is difficult. In addition, the escalating costs of providing care at the end-of-life in acute hospitals are unsustainable. Hospitals in general and emergency departments in particular cannot always provide the best care for patients approaching end-of-life. The main objectives of this paper are to review the existing literature in order to assess the evidence for managing patients dying in the emergency department, and to identify areas of improvement such as supporting different models of care and evaluating those models with health services research. The paper identified six main areas where there is lack of research and/or suboptimal policy implementation. These include uncertainty of treatment in the emergency department; quality of life issues; costs, ethical and social issues; interaction between ED and other health services; and strategies for out of hospital care. The paper concludes with some areas for policy development and future research.

摘要

在急救医疗服务领域，终末期患者的住院及管理方面正对社会构成了严峻挑战，因为大多数临终患者明确表示希望在家中去世，加之从急症护理转到姑息治疗变得十分困难。此外，急症救治医院提供终末期护理的成本不断攀升，具有不可持续性。普通医院，尤其是急诊科往往无法为临近终末期的患者提供最佳护理。本论文的主要目的是回顾现有文献，以评估急诊科管理临终患者的证据，并确定需要改进的方面，如支持不同的护理模式，并通过卫生服务研究评估这些模式。本文确定了缺乏研究或政策实施不理想的六个主要领域，主要包括急诊科治疗的不确定性，生命质量问题，医疗成本、伦理和社会问题，急诊科与其他医疗服务部门的沟通，以及院外临终护理策略。最后，本文提出了一些政策发展和未来研究的领域。

上述摘要先简要叙述了急诊室临终患者住院和管理的一些背景及挑战，重点总结了该文的主要目的是回顾现有文献，评估管理急诊室临终患者的证据，并找出需要改进的地方。该摘要总结了六个主题，最后提出政策制定和未来研究的方向。该摘要只有一段内容，且没有列出关键词。描述性摘要的研究目的常用一般现在时来表达，研究方法和结果常用过去式来表达，结论常用一般现在时来表达。该摘要使用了一般现在时和过去式。

2. 常用表达

（1）The purpose of this literature review is to...

本综述旨在……

（2）This systematic review aims to...

本系统综述旨在……

（3）The objectives of this paper are to review...

本文的目的是梳理 / 回顾……

（4）This paper presents a review of...

本文综述了……

（5）We review...

我们回顾 / 综述了……

（6）The paper identifies...

本文发现……

（7）The paper concludes...

本文总结……

3. 示例

【例 1】

This paper presents a narrative review of the literature on reflection in medical diagnosis aimed at addressing two questions.

本文对医学诊断中反思行为的文献进行了综述，旨在解决两个问题。

【例 2】

The purpose of this literature review is to provide an overview of the information retrieval behavior of clinical nurses, in terms of the use of databases and other information resources and their frequency of use.

该综述旨在概述临床护士群体的信息获取行为，主要涉及数据库和其他信息资源的使用及其使用频率。

【例 3】

This paper identifies the patterns, causes, and control of this disorder in groups of people.

本文发现了某些群体中该疾病的发病模式、病因及控制方法。

10.4.3 引言（Introduction）

1. 内容和要求

引言的目的是帮助读者对所综述的内容形成初步认识，以便引导读者产生进一步阅读全文的兴趣。引言应包括写作目的、有关概念含义、所涉及的内容，扼要介绍有关问题的现状和焦点，为引出正文打下基础。在探讨研究问题和目的时，作者应使用一般现在时。《急诊室临终关怀综述》的英文引言如下所示：

Introduction

Emergency departments (EDs) are increasingly used for patients, whether they are seriously ill as a result of being at the end-of-life (EOL) or whether they have a mainly acute and potentially treatable condition. A growing number of patients at the EOL are admitted to EDs and receive increasingly invasive care. Clinical, social, and economic dimensions have been identified as key aspects of concern.

Studies exploring the impact of hospital care on the quality of the dying process highlight frequent, unsustainable, and sometimes unnecessary costs for an already stressed healthcare system.

There is also evidence that some patients at EOL experience a dying process that not always complies with the basic understanding of a "good death". A comprehensive framework to improve care for the dying was developed by the Institute of Medicine (IOM): "A decent or good death is the one that is: free from avoidable distress and suffering for patients, families, and caregivers; in general accord with patients' and families' wishes; and reasonably consistent with clinical, cultural, and ethical standards." The IOM framework also described several initiatives to improve the care of the dying, but there is limited knowledge about how these models of care for patients at EOL can be applied in the ED.

The main purpose of Emergency Medicine (EM) is to treat undifferentiated patients across age and disease or injury spectra, to create a time-restricted assessment of the patient, to resuscitate and stabilize in order to establish initial or definitive treatment, and finally to discharge the patient to an appropriate facility.

In the case of patients at EOL, these principles cannot always be applied or implemented because these patients cannot be treated in the same manner as patients with no terminal conditions. Secondly, patients at EOL cannot be assessed and treated on the same time-restricted manner as other patients because they often present with multiple complications and several complex conditions. Thirdly, resuscitation and active treatment for these patients may not be the best nor the preferred option, especially if those outcomes are against their wishes, and they cannot always be discharged from ED to an appropriate facility or service.

Of the estimated 140,000 Australians who die each year, it is calculated that at least 100,000 of them die as a result of an "anticipated" or "expected" death. Of the 140,000 who die each year, 54% die in acute care hospitals; 20% die in hospices / palliative care; 16% die at home; 10% die in nursing homes. The elderly tend to be overrepresented in EDs.

The characteristics of patients at EOL comprise a wide range of demographic, clinical, and psychosocial factors in relation to time and places of death. They also comprise a wide range of ages and conditions such as cancer, terminal respiratory diseases, cardiac failure, profound intellectual and physical disability, and advanced dementia. These patients pose a challenge in the ED because the majority appear not to have access to palliative care options, in particular those with non-cancer conditions. Patients are managed in the ED when palliative management at home would have been more appropriate if a transition from active to palliative management had been made earlier.

In the past, the limits of conventional medical treatment were largely determined by the general practitioner (GP). Today, it is more common for the GP to refer the patient to hospital when the illness becomes severe and life is threatened. The GP often faces barriers when managing their patients at EOL making their central role in home-based care difficult. Reasons include unexpected hospitalization contrary to home death as planned as a result of the carer not having sufficient resources and an inability to control unpleasant symptoms. As a result the GP is often bypassed and the patient is admitted to an acute hospital where EDs tend to perform acute resuscitation and transfer to general wards or intensive care units (ICUs).

The following definitions of end of life, end-of-life care, and palliative care, are used throughout this position paper.

(1) End-of-life: It is that part of life where a person is living with, and impaired by, an eventually fatal condition, even if the prognosis is ambiguous or unknown.

(2) End-of-life care: EOL care combines the broad set of health and community services that care for the population at the end of their life. Quality end-of-life care is realized when strong networks exist between specialist palliative care providers, primary generalist providers, primary specialists, and support care providers and the community—working together to meet the needs of the people requiring care.

(3) Palliative care: It is specialist care provided for all people living with, and dying from an eventually fatal condition and for whom the primary goal is quality of life.

In this paper, we discuss the evidence around managing patients at the EOL in the ED setting, in particular some of the clinical, social, ethical, and economic aspects reported in the literature. We also define areas of research and policy development that have not been covered and suggest some potential courses of action.

引言

急诊科正收治越来越多的患者，无论他们是因处于生命终末期而变得病情严重，还是患有急性但有望治愈的疾病。大量的临终患者被送往急诊科接受侵入性治疗。相关的临床、社会和经济方面已成为该领域的主要研究内容。

研究表明，对已经不堪重负的医疗系统来说，医院对临终患者死亡过程的质量护理经常出现不可持续性且有时支出不必要的成本。

还有证据表明，一些处于生命终末期的患者的死亡过程并不总是符合“善终”的理念。（美国）医学研究院制定了一个改善临终关怀的基本框架：“体面的或好的死亡应是：没有对患者、家属和护理人员造成不可避免的痛苦和折磨；总体上符合患者和家属的意愿；并且与临床、文化和伦理标准大体一致。”该框架还描述了若干改善临终关怀的举措，但目前关于这些临终关怀模式如何应用于急诊科，人们了解甚少。

急诊医学的主要目的是治疗不同年龄、患有不同疾病或遭受不同损伤的患者，在有限的时间内评估、抢救和稳定患者病情，以确定初步或最终的治疗方案，最后将患者转移到其他科室或医疗机构治疗。

对于临终患者来说，这些原则并不总是适用或实施，因为这些患者无法和普通患者一样进行相同的治疗。其次，临终患者无法像其他患者那样在有限的时间内进行评估和治疗，因为他们往往伴有多重并发症和复杂病情。第三，复苏和积极治疗可能并不是这些患者的最佳选择，也不是首选，尤其当这些结果与他们的意愿相悖时，且他们无法总是从急诊科被转移到适当的科室或医疗机构治疗。

据估计，每年约有 14 万澳大利亚人死亡，其中至少 10 万人是“可预见”的死亡。在每年死亡的 14 万人中，54% 在急症医院死亡；20% 在临终关怀或姑息治疗机构死亡；16% 死于家中；10% 死于养老院。老年人在急诊科中治疗的比例往往过高。

临终患者的特点包括与时间和死亡地点有关的许多人口统计、临床和心理社会因素。它们包括多个年龄段和多种疾病，如癌症、终末期呼吸道疾病、心力衰竭、严重智力和身体残疾以及晚期痴呆症。这些患者对急诊科构成了挑战，因为大多数人似乎无法获得姑息治疗，尤其是那些患有非癌症疾病的患者。如果能够及早地从积极治疗过渡到姑息治疗，家中可能会更适合，而事实上，患者往往在急诊科接受治疗。

过去，传统医疗的界限主要由全科医生决定。如今，当病情严重且威胁生命时，全科医生常常将患者转诊到医院。全科医生在管理终末期患者时常常面临许多障碍，这使得他们在家庭护理中的核心作用变得困难，因为照护者没有足够的资源、无法控制不适症状，从而造成意外住院，这与计划中在家死亡的理念正好相反。因此，患者常常绕过全科医生这一关被送往急症医院，急诊科进行施救、复苏并转至普通病房或重症监护室。

以下是本文中使用的终末期、终末期护理和姑息治疗的定义。

（1）终末期：终末期是指一个人患有危重病的最后一段时期，即使预后不明确或未知。

（2）终末期护理：终末期护理是指将广泛的健康和社区服务结合在一起，为临终人群提供护理。只有当临终关怀专家、初级全科医生、专科医生、辅助护理人员以及社区之间建立强大网络并相互合作，最终满足患者的需求，才能实现高质量的终末期护理。

（3）姑息治疗：姑息治疗是指为所有患有并将最终死于致命疾病的人提供的专业护理，其主要目标是提高生活质量。

本文讨论了在急诊科管理临终患者的证据，特别是文献中提到的一些临床、社会、伦理和经济方面的问题。我们还定义了尚未涉及的研究和政策发展的领域，并提出了一些可能的行动方案。

该引言篇幅较长，包含多个自然段。其核心是对相关急诊室临终患者研究的背景作初步介绍：越来越多的临终患者去急症科做侵入式治疗。急症科的患者救治具有特殊性，常常和临终患者的治疗原则不一致。因此，临床、社会和经济等方面成了研究热点。该引言还对临终、临终关怀、姑息治疗等术语进行了区分阐释。最后在 Thesis

Statement（论点陈述）部分提出了文献综述的主要内容（见画线部分）：急症科内如何管理临终患者，尤其是涉及临床、社会、伦理和经济方面的问题，还明确提出了政策制定的必要性和未来的研究领域。

2. 常见表达

The aim of the review is to...

本综述旨在……

In the present review of the literature, we intend to...

在目前的文献综述中，我们打算……

In this paper, we discuss the evidence about/around...

本文探讨关于 / 围绕……的证据。

In this systematic review, we will discuss...

本系统综述将探讨……

3. 示例

【例 1】

In this systematic review, we will discuss the evidence on the occurrence of central nervous system (CNS) involvement and neurological manifestations in patients with COVID-19.

本系统综述将讨论新冠患者中枢神经系统及其他神经症状发病率的有关证据。

【例 2】

In the present review of the literature, we intended to contribute to clarify this controversy by addressing two questions.

本综述通过回答两个问题来澄清该争议。

【例 3】

The aim of the review was to identify and synthesize recent studies on the relationship between nurse empowerment and job satisfaction and to make recommendations for further research.

本文对护士赋权与工作满意度的关系进行文献梳理综述，并对未来研究提出建议。

10.4.4 综述方法（Methods of Review）

1. 内容和要求

综述方法部分主要包括下列要素：搜索文献方法、排除与纳入文献的标准、文献数据库来源、研究对象的特征、使用统计分析的情况等。系统综述等类型还需要明确文献搜索的时间范围。研究方法使用一般过去式陈述（见画线部分）。《急诊室临终关怀综述》一文的综述方法如下所示：

Method of Review

We used MEDLINE and EMBASE databases and CareSearch palliative care filter for PubMed to search for articles containing the keywords described in Table 1. Articles were included if they described issues about "terminal care" or "end-of-life" and if they mentioned the "emergency department"; if they explored any "clinical" "social" "ethical", or "economical" issues; or if they referenced "palliative care" or "intensive care" "last year of life" "death", or "dying". We also retrieved relevant grey literature on the topic such as strategic plans and unpublished commissioned research, editorials and policy documents, as well as instruments used in palliative and EOL care. Of the 356 articles indicated in Table 1, 146 articles were rejected on the basis that they did not appear relevant after being screened by title and abstract content. The remaining 210 articles were downloaded, printed, and reviewed for content and quality of evidence. Of these, 50 were excluded as they were not related to ED care. The remaining articles were then sorted using a descriptive thematic approach. We also used SCOPUS to identity the number of citations associated with selected articles.

综述方法

我们使用了（美）联机医学文献分析和检索系统和（荷兰）医学文章数据库以及文献服务检索系统中的临终关怀数据项目筛选，搜索包含表 1 所述关键词的文章。文章被纳入的条件是它们描述了有关“终末期护理”或“生命终期”的问题，并提到了“急诊科”；是否讨论了任何“临床”“社会”“伦理”或“经济”问题；或提到了“临终关怀”“重症监护”“生命的最后一年”“死亡”或“濒死”。我们还收集了该主题的相关灰色文献，如策略计划和未发表的委托研究、社论和政策文件，以及用于临终关怀和生命终末期护理的工具。在表 1 列出的 356 篇文章中，146 篇因在标题和摘要内容筛选后被认为不相关而被排除。剩余的 210 篇文章被下载、打印，并对内容和证据质量审核。在这些文章中，又有 50 篇被排除，因为它们与急诊科护理无关。剩余的文章随后通过描述性主题方法进行分类。我们还使用了斯高帕斯数据库来识别与所选文章相关的引文数量。

该综述方法的作者使用了 MEDLINE、EMBASE、PubMed 等医学论文电子数据库，搜索关键词 terminally ill、terminal care、hospice care、resuscitation orders、withholding treatment、attitude to death、place of death、emergency、emergencies 等确定相关文献。此外，该作者还搜索了相关灰色文献（grey literature，一般指非公开出版的文献）。该作者确定了 356 篇相关文章，再通过题目和摘要内容进一步筛选，排除 146 篇，最后剩下 210 篇文献。经下载、复印和文献阅读后，该作者又剔除 50 篇与急诊科无关联的文章。该作者使用描述性主题法对余下的 160 篇文献进行分类，最后提炼出相关主题进行综合分析。

2. 常用表达

（1）A systematic literature review is performed...

……进行了系统的文献综述。

（2）A comprehensive systematic literature search is carried out according to...

根据……进行了全面、系统的文献检索。

（3）The report of this systematic review is made according to...

本系统综述报告是根据……

（4）The search includes...

搜索包括……

（5）Key search terms include...

主要搜索术语包括……

（6）We search...

我们搜索……（数据库）

（7）We use... to search for...

我们使用……（数据库）搜索……

（8）... fulfill the criteria for inclusion.

……（文章数量）符合纳入标准。

（9）The inclusion criteria for this literature review are as follows...

文献综述的纳入标准如下……

（10）The criteria for exclusion are as follows...

（文献）排除标准如下……

3. 示例

【例 1】

The report of this systematic review was made according to the recommendations of the Preferred Reporting Items for Systematic Reviews and Meta-Analyses (PRISMA) statement.

该系统综述报告以 PRISMA 声明（PRISMA 声明为系统综述和荟萃分析优先报告规范，由 27 个条目组成的清单和一个流程图构成，为系统综述和荟萃分析的规范化撰写和报告提供借鉴和参考）为指导而撰写的。

【例 2】

The search included the following online databases: MEDLINE, CINAHL and SCOPUS.

搜索包括以下网络数据库：联机医学文献分析和检索系统、护理及相关健康文献累积索引和斯高帕斯数据库。

【例 3】

We searched the PubMed and the Web of Science databases for papers published until June 2016 which contained the terms “reflection” “diagnostic reasoning” “reflective reasoning” “critical thinking” “analytic reasoning” “non-analytic reasoning” “pattern-recognition”, and “medical diagnosis” in the title or in the abstract.

我们搜索了 PubMed 和 Web of Science 数据库，搜索时间范围是 2016 年 6 月之前发表的文章，题目或摘要中含有术语“反思”“诊断推理”“反思推理”“批判思维”“分析推理”“非分析推理”“模式识别”和“医学诊断”。

【例 4】

Of 5,272 titles retrieved based on the search strategy, only 9 studies fulfilled the criteria for inclusion.

通过搜索方法搜索到的 5 272 篇文章中，只有 9 篇文献符合纳入标准。

10.4.5 结果（Results）

1. 内容和要求

这一部分是综述的核心部分。系统综述等类型一般分结果和讨论（Results and Discussion）两部分，而传统综述一般直接归纳分析综述的结果。该部分写作方法很多，可因文题大小、内容、所涉及的范围及作者的写作技巧而有所不同。一般常用如下方法：①按选题所属学科的内在科学规律分层阐述，即该学科领域人们的常规思维程序和其间的必然联系；②按目前争论的焦点分别提出问题加以论述的写法；③按学科进展分阶段论述的时间顺序方法；④按临床诊疗工作的程序分述。不管采用何种写作方法，写作内容都应着重论述其历史和现状、发展趋向、各学派的主要观点和争论的焦点、当前研究的新发现和存在的主要问题、对未来发展前景的展望。所引用的资料应确切无误，论据、论证要充分有力，说理应令人信服，客观地反映不同观点，甚至是相反的观点。这部分常使用三种时态：一般过去式、一般现在时、现在完成时。《急诊室临终关怀综述》一文的结果部分如下所示（因篇幅太长，只选取部分内容）：

Results

The thematic analysis identified six main topics of interest, namely, uncertainty of treatment in ED for patients at EOL, quality of life issues, costs, ethical and social issues, interaction between ED and other services, and strategies for out of hospital care.

(1) Uncertainty of Treatment in the Emergency Department for Patients at EOL

O'Connor et al. indicated that in EDs, clinicians often play the role of commencing measures which might be judged to be futile in retrospect, and they argue that the ED environment could be an ideal place for difficult conversations, and difficult decisions regarding withholding of treatment. They also indicated that treatment uncertainty is difficult to measure as it is usually the result of attempting to reach a consensus. Medical futility has been defined both quantitatively by the probability of the success of a treatment and qualitatively by the perceived value in terms of quality of life.

Several articles confirmed that this might be the case in a number of elderly patients with underlying chronic conditions where they may receive active treatment knowing that they will either die in the ED or be admitted by hospital staff knowing that they would die in the near future. Reasons for these actions have been associated with miscommunications between doctors and patients; carers and patients, and between health care staff, and lack of information or cultural factors.

Prognostication based on symptom characteristics such as recurrent infections, weight loss, falls, and functional decline has been used in predicting end-stage disease. Specific symptoms of certain conditions such as ovarian carcinoma have specifically been associated with shorter survival times, namely, bone marrow depression, renal failure, and dyspnoea. Validation studies related to basic life support have been conducted to identify patients with no probability of survival. One study found that following rules for the termination of basic life support had a positive predictive value for death of 99.5% and decreased the transfer of patients to hospital by 63%.

The review also found that the reliability of prognostic models by critical care specialists and ED physicians regarding impending mortality of patients with poor functional outcome is not consistent. In a six-month follow-up study, the reliability of prognosis had a low sensitivity of 35%–37% suggesting that only one third of people with poor prognosis were likely to die. In addition, they had a very high specificity of 99% and positive predictive values of 96%, suggesting that most people expected to live survived (only 1% die when they were expected to live).

In summary, this review found that clinicians in the ED confront a major dilemma about uncertainty of treatment. The dilemma is whether an accurate prediction of appropriate active treatment is possible and whether decisions about a transition to palliation can be made.

(2) Quality of Life Issues

...

(3) Costs

...

(4) Ethical and Social Issues

...

(5) Interaction between ED and Other Health Services

...

(6) Strategies for out of Hospital Care

...

研究结果

本研究通过主题分析的研究方法确定了六个主要感兴趣的议题，即急诊科临终患者治疗的不确定性、生命质量问题、医疗成本、伦理和其他社会问题、急诊科与其他科室的沟通问题以及院外临终护理的策略问题。

（1）急诊科临终患者治疗的不确定性

奥康纳等人指出，急诊科医生经常采用紧急治疗的方案，而这些方案在就诊后经常被认为是徒劳的。他们认为，急诊科是进行艰难对话和做出停止治疗决定的理想场所。他们还指出，很难衡量治疗方案的不确定性，因为治疗方案通常是多方努力达成的共识。无效医疗的定义既包含定量，也涉及定性方面的内容，定量指的是治疗成功的可能性，定性则是患者对生活质量方面的自我感知。

一些文章证实，对于一些患有潜在慢性病的老年人而言，他们可能会在明知自己会死在急诊科，或者被医务人员告知会在短时间内死亡的情况下，仍然选择接受积极治疗。这一现象主要是和医患、护患、医护内部沟通不足，以及信息或者文化层面知识匮乏有关。

症状特征（如重复感染、体重减轻、跌打损伤和功能衰退）已被用于预测终末期疾病的结局。例如，卵巢癌会伴随有骨髓抑制、肾衰竭和呼吸困难等症状，这常与患者存活期较短有关。研究人员已经开展了与基础生命支持措施相关的研究，从而验证无生存希望的患者的实际存活率。一项研究发现，遵循终止基础生命支持的规则，死亡阳性预测值高达 99.5%，减少了 63% 的患者转移到医院。

本综述还发现，重症监护专业人员和急诊科医生针对濒死患者死亡的预后模型可靠性评价并不一致。在一项为期六个月的随访研究中，预后可靠性的灵敏度较低，仅为 35%～37%，这表明只有 1/3 的预后不良患者可能会死亡。此外，他们的特异性高达 99%，阳性预测值为 96%，这表明大多数预期存活的患者都幸存了下来（仅有 1% 的患者在预期会存活的情况下死亡）。

总之，本研究发现急诊科医生面临着医疗方案不确定性的重大困境，这一困境在于能否迅速启动精准有效的治疗方案，以及能否做出向安宁治疗过渡的临床决策。

（2）生命质量问题

……

（3）医疗成本

……

（4）伦理和社会问题

……

（5）急诊科与其他科室的沟通

……

（6）院外临终护理的策略问题

……

本文结果部分开头对相关文献进行文献引用率汇总（因该部分不常见，探讨省略），然后对文献进行分析并总结为六个主题（见第一处画线部分）：①急诊室临终患者治疗的不确定性；②生命质量问题；③费用问题；④伦理和社会问题；⑤急诊室和其他科室的沟通；⑥院外临终护理的策略方法。随后，本文对这六点内容分别进行论述。在第一个主题“急诊室临终患者治疗的不确定性”中，作者通过引用文献分别从几个小层次进行阐述，先阐述了奥康纳（O’Connor）等人的研究成果，急诊室医生在治疗临终患者时通常是无效果的（不管是治疗成功的概率还是生命质量的提高）；接着提及其他几项研究，证实很多有慢性基础性疾病的老年人，尽管明知自己即将死去，但仍然接受了积极治疗，这主要是医生和患者、看护者和患者沟通不畅等原因造成的；然后又引证了其他一些研究，涉及基于一些临床症状可以精确预测的晚期疾病。但还有些研究发现急症科专家对一些预后较差的患者的预测并不准确。最后是一个小结：急症科医生对于是为临终患者做出准确预测进行积极治疗，还是将患者转到临终关怀机构而左右为难。

2. 常见表达

（1）The thematic analysis identifies...

主题分析表明……

（2）... themes are identified...

……发现了……主题。

（3）To summarize the results of the review, we will group the papers according to...

为了总结综述结果，我们根据……将论文分类。

（4）The review also finds...

本综述发现了……

（5）... indicates that...

……表明……

（6）Several articles confirm that...

多篇文章证实……

（7）The results of this study suggest that...

本研究结果表明……

（8）... are summarized in...

……总结了……

（9）... shows the summary of...

……总结……

（10）... examines the relationship...

……探讨了……关系。

3. 示例

【例 1】

Through meta-synthesis, three key themes were identified: ① emotional impact of pediatric EOL (end of life) care and death, ② perspective of delivering optimal care: what works and what does not, and ③ the complex role of nurses in pediatric EOL care.

通过荟萃分析，发现了三个主题：①儿科临终关怀和死亡的情感影响；②实施最优护理的论述：包括有效的和无效的护理；③儿科临终关怀护士的复杂角色。

【例 2】

The results of this study suggested that the negative relation between nurse empowerment and job strain is consistent with both Kanter's and Karasek's theories.

这项研究结果表明护士授权和工作压力呈负相关，与坎特及卡拉赛克理论一致。

【例 3】

Ahmad and Oryane found that there are differences in the relationship between empowerment and commitment among nurses who come from two different cultural contexts: Malaysia and England.

阿哈默德和奥瑞恩发现来自马来西亚和英国不同文化背景的护士授权与承诺之间的关系存在差异。

【例 4】

The characteristics of the studies included in this review are summarized in Tables 2 and 3.

表 2 和表 3 总结了本综述中文献呈现出的特点。

【例 5】

Table 3 shows the summary of these studies on the central nervous system (CNS) manifestations of COVID-19.

表 3 总结了新冠（患者）中枢神经系统症状的研究。

10.4.6 结论（Conclusion）

1. 内容和要求

结论概括正文部分的主要内容。研究者在这一部分最好能提出自己的见解，如赞成什么、反对什么、今后应注重发展什么等。结论部分常用一般现在时和一般将来时。《急诊室临终关怀综述》一文的结论部分如下所示：

Summary and Conclusions

As patients approach EOL, their disease process may create an immediate life-threatening emergency normally requiring admission to an ED, yet further active treatment is futile. A large number of elderly patients at EOL die in the ED and many of them are admitted to hospital knowing that they are dying and that modern interventional medicine has little to offer.

As indicated at the beginning, the main purpose of EM is to treat undifferentiated patients across age and disease or injury spectra, to create a time-restricted assessment of the patient, to resuscitate and stabilize in order to establish initial or definitive treatment, and finally to discharge the patient to an appropriate facility. As unraveled in this paper, these principles are not always possible to implement exactly as prescribed when managing patients facing EOL. Organizing the most appropriate care for these patients can be time-consuming, requiring honest and timely prognostic information, clear recommendations, facilitating patient-family discussions, and affirming patient choices.

The following is a list of policy and practice recommendations and discussion of the need for further research derived from the findings of this review.

(1) Better Prognostic Models

The reliability of estimating death for patients with poor functional outcomes is low. Treatment futility is also difficult to prognosticate and is complicated by variation of what may be perceived as an acceptable probability of success but an unacceptable level of quality of life or vice versa. More precise instruments with higher sensitivity to assess EOL timelines in the ED are needed. That knowledge could be used to offer a timely transition from active treatment to palliative care with the suspension of futile care in the ED.

(2) Specialized Training

...

(3) A Structured Approach to Decision-Making

...

(4) Infrastructure, Information, and Planning Ahead

...

(5) Evidence-Based Research About EOL Care in the ED

...

Furthermore, the patterns of life, disease, dying, and death have changed dramatically in recent years across the world, and research is essential to develop evidence-based public health policy. Further research should include evaluation of pathways for the appropriate care of terminal patients in the ED (such as the LCP), and comparison of services across countries such as the UK where GPs are required to do home visits on sick people and are financially penalized for hospital admissions and Australia, where this is not the case. Finally, we support the identification of robust rules for patients receiving inappropriate advanced life support care.

总结

当患者生命临近终末期时，他们的病程可能会突发危及生命的紧急情况，通常需要入住急诊科进行积极治疗，但往往是徒劳的。许多老年临终患者死于急症科，其中许多患者在入院时就知道自己时日无多，现代医学介入几乎无能为力。

如开头所述，急诊医学的主要目的是治疗不同年龄、患有不同疾病或遭受不同损伤的患者，在有限的时间内评估、抢救和稳定患者病情，从而确定初步或最终治疗方案，最后将患者转移到适当的医疗机构治疗。正如本文所揭示的那样，在照顾面临临终关怀的患者时，医生并不总能够严格按照规定实施医学行为。为这类患者安排最合适的护理方式可能会耗费大量时间，需要及时提供真实的预后信息、明确的诊疗意见，还需要促进患者与家属的沟通，并且确认患者自己的选择。

以下是从本综述结果中得出的政策和实践建议，以及未来研究需要的讨论。

（1）（建立）更好的预后模型

对于功能不良患者的死亡预期估计可靠性较低。很难评估预后何为无效治疗，原因在于患者可以接受的成功率和不可接受的生活质量的变化而变得复杂，反之亦然。我们需要灵敏度更高、精准度更高的工具来评估临终患者的存活期，这些知识和工具储备有助于医生及时从积极治疗过渡到安宁治疗，并且停止无效的急诊治疗。

（2）（开展）专业培训

……

（3）（实施）结构化的决策策略

……

（4）（优化医疗）基础设施，（实现医疗）信息化和提前规划

……

（5）（开展）急诊医学有关的临终关怀循证研究

……

此外，近年来，世界各地的生活、疾病、临终和死亡模式都发生了巨大变化，因此开展研究对于制定循证公共卫生政策至关重要。后续研究应包括评估急救医学中临终患者适合的护理路径，比较不同国家的医疗服务，如英国和澳大利亚，前者要求全科医生对病患定期家访，还会因病患入院而罚款，而后者并没有这项制度。最后，我们支持明确的规则，规定哪些患者不适合接受生命急救护理。

本文结论部分前两段概括了综述的核心内容：许多临终患者都会出现紧急的状况，

通常需要进入急症科抢救，然而进一步的积极治疗通常是无效的。许多处于临终期的老年人明知即将离开世界还是接受住院治疗，现代医学对其无能为力。急症医学的目的是对一切危重患者进行及时评估、救治，然后将患者转入其他合适的科室。但是，应对临终患者时，这些原则并不总能有效准确地实施。为临终患者安排最合适的治疗很耗时，不仅需要医生坦诚的预后信息、明确的建议，还需要患者和家庭成员之间的有效沟通以及患者自己的抉择。此外，作者还提出了六项政策和医疗实践建议，以及对该问题进一步研究探讨的必要性。

2. 常用表达

（1）Further research should include...

进一步研究应包括……

（2）We recommend that...

我们建议……

（3）... is recommended...

建议……

（4）The findings of this review provide evidence of...

本综述的发现提供了……证据。

（5）This review could be useful to...

本综述可对……有用。

3. 示例

【例 1】

Further research on this topic is recommended, and particularly studies from Europe and Australia are needed.

建议对这一主题进行进一步研究，尤其需要来自欧洲和澳大利亚的相关研究。

【例 2】

The findings of this review provide evidence of the importance of workplace empowerment to achieve positive organizational outcomes in nursing.

本综述的发现为护理工作授权以获取良好的组织结果的重要性提供了依据。

【例 3】

This review could be useful to guide leaders' strategies to develop and maintain empowering work, so enhancing job satisfaction, in turn leading to nurse retention and positive patient outcomes.

本综述可能有助于指导领导者制定和维持授权工作的策略，能够提高护士工作满意度，鼓励护士留任，提升患者护理效果。

10.4.7 文献（References）

参考文献是医学文献综述论文的重要组成部分，不能省略。引用文献的多寡是判断综述质量好坏的一个标志。参考文献是文献综述写作的重要依据，也为阅读者提供了寻找原始论文的线索，也是对原始论文作者的劳动尊重的表示。

参考文献一般引自公开出版、发表的图书、杂志等，文中一定要标注。参考文献格式按期刊的具体要求来呈现。参考文献的数量不一，多者可上千篇，少者几十篇。《急诊室临终关怀综述》一文列出的文献有 162 篇。

10.5 综述语言特征（Language Features of Literature Review）

10.5.1 转述动词（Reporting Verb）的使用

文献综述的一个主要语言特征是使用转述动词。转述动词用于描述或汇报相关文献，可以表明作者对他人研究的态度，持赞成、反对或中立的立场。例如，描述研究目的常用 investigate、examine、look at 等，.论述研究结果常用 show、suggest、reveal 等，展示某人的观点常用 state、believe、argue 等。其他常用的转述动词（短语）还有：adapt、arise、confirm、clarify、demonstrate、determine、establish、exhibit、focus on、feel、generate、hold、identify、manifest、propose、prove、recognize、reveal、verify、write 等。

10.5.2 评估性和谨慎语言（Evaluative and Cautious Language）的使用

文献综述中，作者可以使用评估性语言表明自己对他人研究观点的态度，可以赞成，也可以反对。赞同他人观点的常用词语有 convincing、crucial、effective、necessary 等；反对的常用词语有 questionable、unclear、inconclusive、trivial 等。此外，表达肯定语气时，作者还常使用增强语（boosters），常见的词语有：accurately、clearly、certainly、definitely、without a doubt、unquestionably；常见的句型有：It is certain...、It is highly possible...、It is widely agreed...、There is strong evidence...。谨慎语（cautious language）是指在可能存在不确定的情况下，对表达肯定话语的谨慎使用。模糊限制语（hedges）就是一种谨慎语言，表明不确定的态度。常见的词语有：appear to、seem、possibly、likely、somewhat、suggest、may mean、would require；常见的句型有：The project is likely to...、It may be...、If Malouf's (2021) findings are...、There is some evidence...。

Exercises

Exercise I Answer the following questions.

1. How long should an abstract be?
2. Can you list at least five hedges used in the literature review?
3. Can you list at least three databases associated with medical research?

Exercise II Conduct a literature search of the recent development about traditional Chinese medicine (TCM) to treat advanced lung cancer.

Exercise III Based on the literature search in Exercise II, write a method of review.

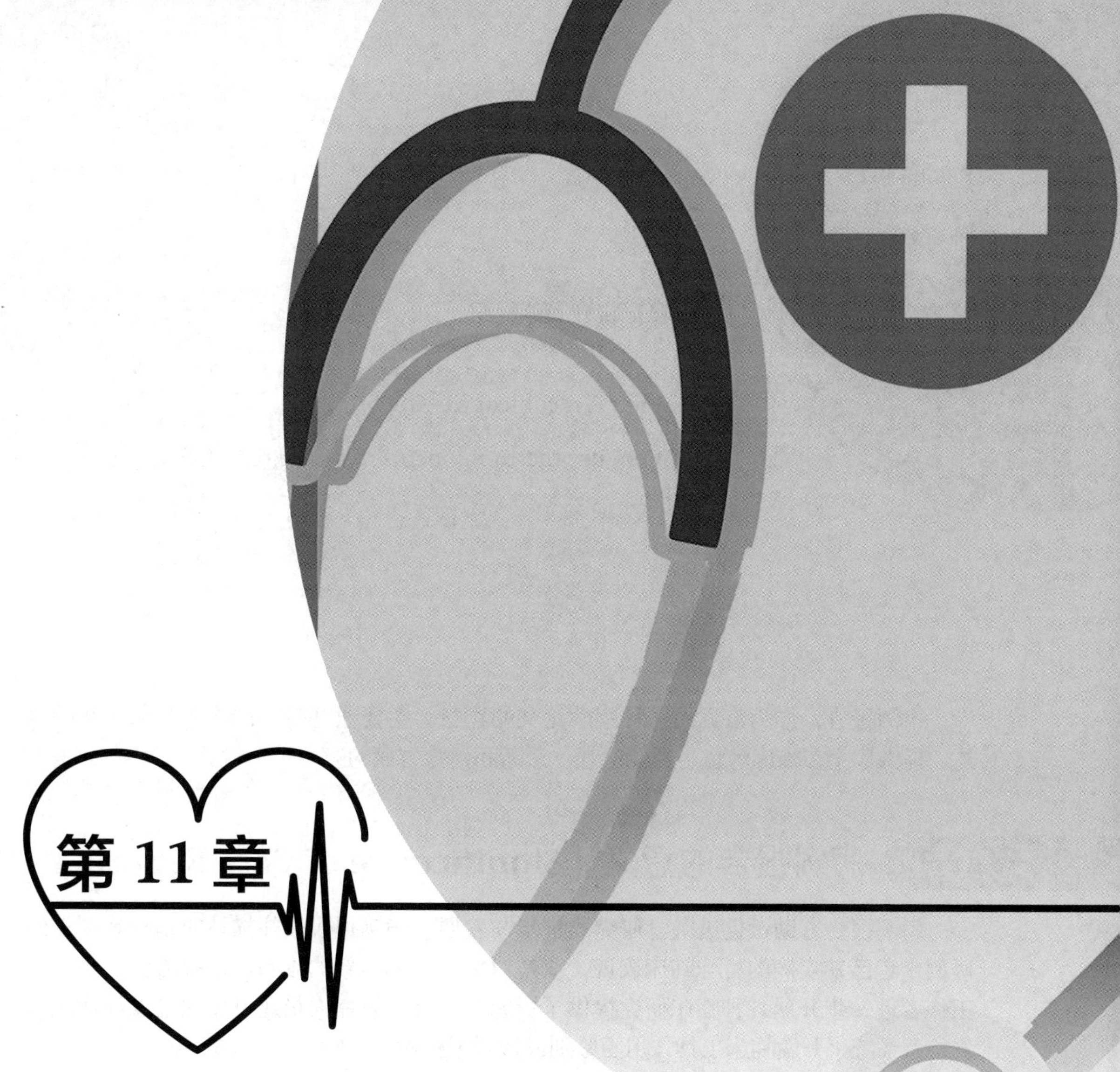

第 11 章

病例报告
（Case Reports）

Diseases come on horseback but steal away on foot.

病来如山倒，病去如抽丝。

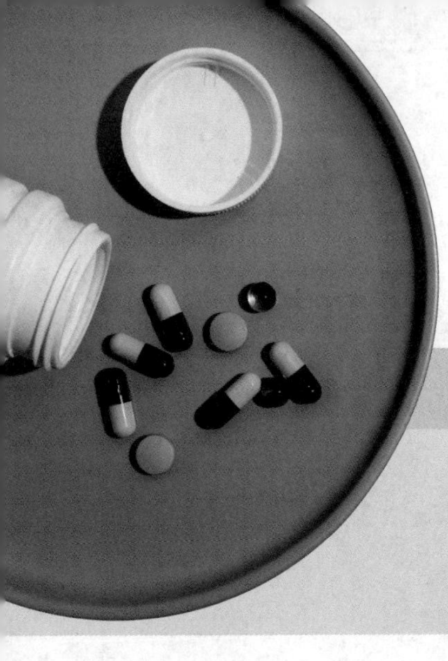

Warm-up

1. What is a clinical case report?
2. What are the components of a case report?

病例报告，作为常见的一种医学论文的题材，主要通过对一例或者几例病案的描述，提供病案在临床症状、影像检查、诊断和治疗方面的第一手资料。

11.1 病例报告的意义（Significance of Case Reports）

病例报告有助于促进医学研究的进步与发展。病例报告往往描述的是较为罕见的病例或者已知疾病的特殊临床表现，或是对常见病例的新的诊断与治疗方法，为医学工作者进一步开展各种临床研究提供了资源。此外，研究人员还可以通过设计病例报告检索系统来开发临床工具，用于鉴别或诊断某些病症。

11.2 病例报告的范围（Scope of Case Reports）

病例报告通常分为以下几类：

（1）罕见病例；

（2）疾病的异常表现或异常组合；

（3）困难诊断或者无定论诊断；

（4）治疗或管理方面的难题；

（5）对疾病或病症的新见解的观察等。

11.3 病例报告的构成（Composition of Case Reports）

病例报告通常由标题（Title）、摘要（Abstract）、引言（Introduction）、病例描述

（Case Report）、讨论（Discussion/Comment）和结论（Conclusion）组成。有的病例报告还附有图表（Graphs and Illustrations）以及参考文献（References）。本章重点讨论最重要的三个部分——引言、病例描述和讨论的写作方法。

11.3.1 引言（Introduction）

病例报告的引言主要对病例的特殊性以及选取病例的意义进行解释和说明。引言部分一般使用一般现在时。

1. 常用表达

1）阐述病例报告的目的

- This article is designed to point out some of the possible pitfalls...
  本文旨在指出一些可能出现的陷阱……
- To the best of our knowledge, this is the first reported case of...
  据我们所知，这是第一例……的报告病例。

2）简要描述病例

- We present a case of...
  我们在此介绍一例……
- The present case describes...
  本病例描述……

2. 示例

【例 1】

Trigeminal neuralgia (TN) is generally caused by vascular compression of the nerve root. Cerebellopontine angle (CPA) tumors might also sometimes provoke TN by directly compressing the trigeminal nerve root or indirectly by displacing arteries. In such cases, the tumors are usually large enough to be diagnosed radiographically. We present herein a case of TN caused by a very small meningioma covering the suprameatal tubercle that displayed hyperostosis at the entrance of Meckel's cave and was not obvious on routine magnetic resonance (MR) images.

三叉神经痛通常是由神经根的血管压迫引起的。小脑桥脑角肿瘤有时也可能通过直接压迫三叉神经根或通过置换动脉间接引起三叉神经痛。通常在这种情况下，肿瘤体积足够大，可以通过放射成像进行诊断。我们在此介绍一例由覆盖在膈上结节的非常小的脑膜瘤引起的三叉神经痛病例，该脑膜瘤在梅克尔腔入口处显示为骨质增生，并且在常规磁共振图像上并不明显。

【例 2】

Conjunctival amyloid is a well-documented albeit rare condition although at least 40 cases have been reported in the literature. Localized conjunctival amyloidosis may be primary or secondary. In the primary type no underlying disease of the conjunctiva is present, whereas secondary localized amyloidosis of the conjunctiva has been reported in association with trachoma and recurrent bacterial conjunctivitis. More rarely, conjunctival amyloid may be part of primary systemic amyloidosis, but the conjunctiva is usually spared in secondary systemic amyloidosis. The present case describes primary localized amyloidosis of the conjunctiva in which the amyloid was characterized as AL (immunoglobulin-derived) by histochemistry and immunocytochemistry.

结膜淀粉样蛋白是一种有据可查但较为罕见的疾病，尽管有至少 40 例相关文献报道。局限性结膜淀粉样变性可分为原发性或继发性两种类型。原发性类型未呈现结膜的潜在疾病，而继发性局限性淀粉样变性则与沙眼和复发性细菌性结膜炎有关。更为罕见的是，结膜淀粉样蛋白可能是原发性系统性淀粉样变性的一部分，但在继发性系统性淀粉样变性中结膜却未呈现。本病例描述了结膜的原发性局限性淀粉样变性，组织化学和免疫细胞化学认为其特征为轻链淀粉样变性（免疫球蛋白衍生）。

11.3.2 病例描述（Case Presentation）

病例描述部分对病例的病史、检查、诊断与治疗以及治疗结果进行充分的描述。病例描述一般为正叙法，使用一般现在时。描述应保持客观，清楚准确地说明患者整个病程的情况，同时应突出病例的罕见性或突出其特殊意义。

1. 病史

病史（Case History）通常包括病例的年龄、性别、发病时间、发病经过、主诉及家族病史等情况。

1）常用表达

（1）描述患者的基本情况，如年龄、性别、身高、体重、种族和职业等信息

- A(n)... -year-old man/woman is admitted to hospital with...

  患者为……岁男性 / 女性，因……收治入院。

- A(n)... -year-old man/woman presents with...

  患者为……岁男性 / 女性，症状表现为……

（2）描述患者的既往病史、生活习惯或家族病史

- He has been hypertensive for 10 years.

  他患有高血压长达 10 年。

- In addition, she has a 5-year history of difficulty with swallowing.
  此外，她有五年的吞咽困难史。
- There is no family history of renal disease.
  无肾脏疾病家族史。

2）示例

【例 1】

A 55-year-old woman presented as a thrombolysis call, with a sudden onset of abnormal, involuntary movements affecting her left arm and leg and a left-sided facial droop. She had a 2-day history of left-sided stiffness. Her previous history included type 2 diabetes mellitus, hypertension, hypercholesterolemia, and chronic depression. Her diabetic control had recently worsened due to self-neglect. She had never smoked and did not drink alcohol.

患者为 55 岁女性，因溶栓就诊，左臂和左腿出现突然的异常、不自主运动以及左侧面部下垂。她有两天的左侧僵硬病史。既往病史包括 II 型糖尿病、高血压、高胆固醇血症和慢性抑郁症。由于自我忽视，其糖尿病控制最近恶化。无吸烟、饮酒史。

【例 2】

A 26-year-old builder's laborer presented to the A&E Department of the Luton and Dunstable Hospital having been stung approximately 30 minutes previously by a bee in the posterior triangle of the right side of the neck. He complained of weakness and tingling sensations in the right upper limb but no other neurological symptoms. He was otherwise fit and well.

一名 26 岁的建筑工人被送往卢顿和邓斯特布尔医院的急诊部。他在大约 30 分钟前被一只蜜蜂蜇伤右侧颈后三角。主诉右上肢无力和刺痛感，无其他神经系统症状。除此之外，无异常情况。

2. 检查

检查（Physical Examination）部分应报告有意义的阳性结果和有意义的阴性结果。检查部分往往需要附上检查结果的报告或图表。

1）常用表达

（1）描述体格检查结果

- No other joint appears to be affected.
  其他关节无影响。
- His pulse is .../min and regular. His blood pressure is .../... mmHg. Examination of his heart, chest, and abdomen is normal.

患者脉搏正常，为每分钟……次。血压为……毫米汞柱。心脏、胸部和腹部检查均为正常。

（2）报告检查结果

- A cytological examination of the ulcers showed...
  溃疡的细胞学检查显示……
- On examination the patient was seen to have...
  经检查，发现患者有……
- Radiographs showed... (Fig. 3). Sialography of... normal.
  射线照片显示……（图 3）。……唾液造影正常。

2）示例

【例 1】

On examination, her temperature is 37.5°C. Her pulse rate is 120/min and regular. Blood pressure is 90/70 mmHg. Jugular venous pressure is raised at 8 cm. On auscultation, there is a gallop rhythm, with a third heart sound. Examination of her chest is unremarkable. Pressure over the sternum causes discomfort. Abdominal and neurological examination is normal.

经检查，她的体温为 37.5 摄氏度，脉率为 120/分钟，律规整。血压为 90/70 毫米汞柱。颈静脉压升高至 8 厘米。听诊时，有奔马律，伴有第三心音。胸部检查无明显异常。胸骨受压会引起不适。腹部和神经系统检查正常。

【例 2】

Biochemical investigations were performed and the results are illustrated in Table 1. Additionally, CXR, ECG, FBC, ESR, prothrombin time, alkaline phosphatase and thyroid function tests were normal.

生化检查结果见表 1。此外，胸部 X 光片检查、心电图、全血细胞计数、红细胞沉降率、凝血酶原时间、碱性磷酸酶和甲状腺功能测试均正常。

3. 诊断与治疗

诊断与治疗（Diagnosis and Treatment）部分包括诊断的依据、治疗的方案、步骤过程及使用的药物等信息。诊断部分可以阐明微生物学、超声检查等医学影像结果以及各种血清学、病理学、免疫学等方面的测试结果，以作为诊断的基础。治疗部分应该给出所有治疗、给药剂量、给药途径和治疗间隔的完整信息。

1）常用表达

（1）描述做出诊断

- A diagnosis of... is made. / ... is diagnosed as...
  被诊断为……

- The definitive diagnosis was made after surgical excision.

  手术切除后做出明确诊断。

（2）描述治疗过程

- Initial treatment of... includes therapeutic thoracentesis for relief of...

  ……的初始治疗包括治疗性胸腔穿刺术，以缓解……

- The patient was treated initially with...

  患者最初接受……治疗。

- After a full course of...

  经过一个完整的……疗程之后……

2）示例

【例 1】

The hepatitis A resolved after three weeks of restricted physical activity. We soaped the wound three times a day and administered sulphamethizole 2 g twice a day for 14 days.

甲型肝炎在限制患者身体活动三周后消退。我们每天三次用肥皂对患者的伤口进行消毒，患者每天服用磺胺甲唑两次，每次 2 克，持续 14 天。

【例 2】

Echocardiography revealed the presence of bicuspid aortic valves and vegetations attached to both the cusps dangling in the left ventricular outflow tract during diastole. Hence, the diagnosis of infective endocarditis was made on the basis of Duke's criteria. The patient was treated with a course of antibiotics comprising ceftriaxone 3 g/day and amikacin 15 mg/kg body weight for a period of two weeks, followed by ceftriaxone 3 g/day for the next two weeks.

超声心动图显示存在二叶式主动脉瓣，并且在舒张期时，两个瓣叶上都有赘生物悬挂在左心室流出道中。因此，根据杜克标准，诊断为感染性心内膜炎。患者接受一个疗程的抗生素治疗，包括头孢曲松 3 克 / 天，以及按照每千克体重 15 毫克使用阿米卡星，为期两周。随后两周使用头孢曲松 3 克 / 天。

4. 治疗结果

治疗结果（Outcome）部分应对治疗结束时临床病症的消退程度以及之后的随访等进行详细说明。

1）常用表达

- She was discharged... days later without any complications.

  她……天后出院，无任何并发症。

- The patient is still monitored regularly, currently with normal... laboratory findings.

  患者仍接受定期监测，目前，……实验室检查结果正常。

2）示例

【例 1】

The cyst was successfully excised and sent for histopathologic analysis. There were no intraoperative or immediate postprocedure complications. The patient was discharged home on the day of surgery.

成功切除囊肿并将其送去做组织病理分析。无术中或术后并发症。患者于手术当天出院。

【例 2】

She showed marked improvement of proptosis and orbital congestion, but limitations in extraocular movements persisted.

患者眼球突出和眼眶充血的状况有明显改善，但眼外运动仍然受限。

11.3.3 讨论（Discussion）

讨论部分应对病例的罕见性或特殊意义进行论述，证明病例的独特性。如所描述病例在文献中已有类似病例，作者应指出该病例与已有病例的不同之处。同时，讨论部分应对下一步的研究提出建议。

1. 常用表达

- We suggest that... should be included among the differential diagnosis in...

  我们建议应将……纳入对……的鉴别诊断中。

- This case highlights the importance of..., and the need to investigate further...

  本病例凸显了……的重要性，以及进一步调查……的必要性。

2. 示例

【例 1】

The correct diagnosis of pelvic pain with the possibility of ruptured ectopic pregnancy is very challenging. The patient with a history of tubal surgery and few weeks of amenorrhea and vaginal bleeding is the typical picture of an ectopic pregnancy. The pelvic ultrasound is helpful but we can get better results with a vaginal probe ultrasound. Also, the follow-up of quantitative HCG is important. The patient was immediately prepared for laparoscopic surgery, possible laparotomy. The patient underwent a laparoscopic salpingostomy on the right tube.

盆腔疼痛和异位妊娠破裂可能性的正确诊断非常具有挑战性。异位妊娠的典型特征为患者有输卵管手术史以及数周闭经和阴道出血。骨盆超声检查有帮助，但可以通过阴道探头超声检查获得更好的结果。此外，定量人体绒毛膜促性腺激素的随访也很重要。患者立即准备进行腹腔镜手术，并有可能需要进行剖腹术。患者接受了右侧输卵管的腹腔镜造口术。

【例 2】

Ursodeoxycholic acid is used to slow down the progression of the disease with mixed reports as to whether they improve mortality. Other treatments involve altering the autoimmune component of the condition with methotrexate, for example. Transplant is also an option; however, the autoimmune process affects the transplanted liver and other problems such as rejection are likely.

熊去氧胆酸被用于减缓疾病的进展，但关于其是否能改善生存率的报道结果不一。其他治疗方法，如使用甲氨蝶呤，在于改变疾病的自身免疫成份。移植也是一种选择，但是自身免疫过程会影响移植的肝脏，并且还可能出现诸如排斥反应等问题。

Exercises

Exercise I　Choose the correct answer for the following questions.

1. When are case reports most useful?

A) When practice guidelines are developed.

B) When the population being studied is very large.

C) When new symptoms or outcomes are unidentified.

D) When you encounter common cases and need more information.

2. Which of the following is unrelated to the case presentation?

A) Description of the patient's complaint.

B) Patient's medical/family/social history.

C) The uniqueness and significance of the case.

D) Pertinent findings on the patient's physical examination.

Exercise II Judge whether each of the following statements is true or false. Put T for true or F for false in the brackets.

1. The patient should be described in detail, allowing others to identify patients with similar characteristics in a case report. (   )
2. Case reports are based on systematic studies and surely can be generalized. (   )
3. Case reports should include carefully recorded, unbiased observations. (   )
4. The patient's diet history ought to be included in the case report. (   )

Exercise III Translate the following paragraphs into Chinese.

1. We report the case of a man in his 40s who was referred to the ear, nose, and throat outpatient department by a regional emergency department with a 12-month history of nasal swelling. The swelling had gradually increased in size since the onset, causing symptoms of pain and right-sided nasal blockage. There was no associated discharge from the swelling. The patient did not report rhinorrhea or anosmia and had no red-flag symptoms.
2. On examination, she has a blood pressure of 102/65 mmHg and a pulse of 78/min which is regular. The heart sounds are normal. There is some tenderness on the left side of the chest, to the left of the sternum and in the left submammary area. The respiratory rate is 22/min. No abnormalities were found on examination of the lungs. She is tender in the left iliac fossa.
3. Our case shows the importance of medical and microbiological services collaborating adequately. When submitting specimens for microbiological investigations from patients who have been abroad, clinicians should give the relevant geographical information.

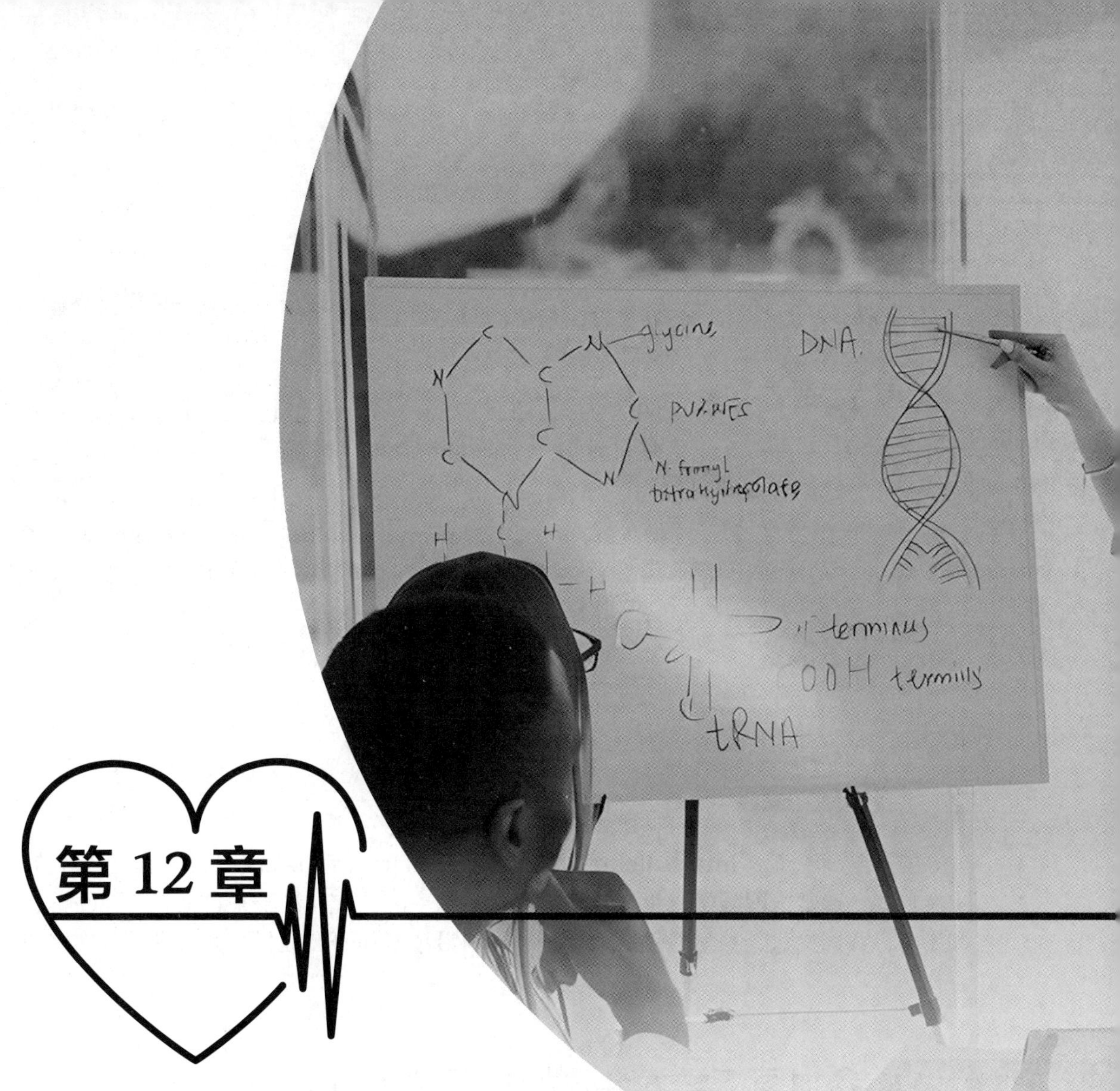

第 12 章

国际医学会议（International Medical Conferences）

If you have an apple and I have an apple, and we exchange apples, we both still only have one apple. But if you have an idea and I have an idea, and we exchange ideas, we each now have two ideas.

你有一个苹果，我有一个苹果，我们交换一下，一人还是只有一个苹果；你有一个想法，我有一个想法，我们交换一下，一人就有两个想法。

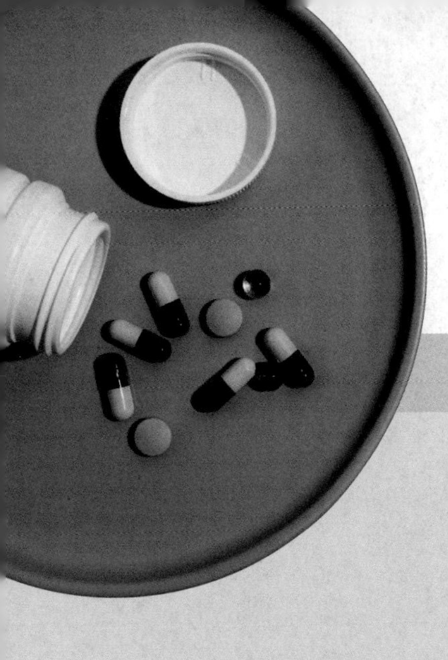

Warm-up

1. When you want to apply for an international conference, what should you do to prepare?
2. What contents will you report when you are invited to give a speech in an international academic conference? Say, research background, methods, results, and other key elements of your research.

国际学术会议（International Academic Conference，IAC）是一种学界交流的重要形式，通常由国际学术组织或相关学术机构主办，旨在汇集来自世界各地的学者和专家，共同探讨某一学科领域的新进展、前沿技术和研究成果，并促进学术交流和合作。

12.1 参加国际学术会议的重要性（Importance of Attending IAC）

国际学术会议是加强学生国际化培养、促进高校教育国际化的重要途径。参加国际会议具有以下重要价值：第一，有利于了解该学术领域国际研究发展最新状况与发展趋势，开阔视野。第二，有利于提升跨文化沟通能力和国际活动能力，提高学术英语水平。第三，通过与领域内学术造诣较深的学者和专家交流，可以提高学术起点，拓宽学术交流与沟通的渠道，有利于今后科研工作的开展。第四，通过参加学术会议，学生还可以了解举办学术会议的一般流程，为今后组织学术会议积累经验。第五，通过大会报告及发言，可加深国内外专家对参会者所在的学科和院校的了解，促进院校的国际化交流。第六，通过参加国际会议，可以明确自己的研究现状与发展前沿的差距，并有效利用会议信息取长补短，做出改进。

12.2 会议通知（Conference Notice）

1. 内容和要求

在举办一项国际学术会议之前，主办方需要先成立会议组委会，制订会议计划并发布会议通知，吸引相关研究领域的学者申请参会。在申请参会之前，学者首先需要阅读会议通知，然后根据通知内容递交参会申请。会议通知由会议主办方的官方网站发布，通常分为简要的征稿通知（Call for Papers）和详细的会议通知（Conference Notice）两种形式。简要的征稿通知主要介绍会议论文征集的主题、格式和要求，会议的时间和地点，投稿方式（如邮箱投稿或官网系统投稿）等；详细的会议通知在此基础上，还会包含会议召开的目的、背景和主题，组织机构和委员会介绍，邀请的与会者，申请参会的资格，会议的组织方，会议日程，参会的登记与接待工作等。

2. 示例

会议通知

下面以美国心理健康研究学会（American Association of Mental Health，AAMH）2022 年发布的会议通知为例，了解国际学术会议的通知内容。同时，此次会议的投稿是通过 AAS 官网系统进行的，对投稿要求做出了详细规定，有助于学生学习规范的会议投稿须知。

Dear Community:

We are excited to announce the Call for Abstracts for AAS22—the 55th Annual Conference of the American Association of Mental Health! The activities are organized in a hybrid format with a dynamic in-person conference and a virtual attendance option. AAS22 will be held April 28–30, 2022 at the Hyatt Regency O'Hare in Chicago, as well as online, with pre-conference workshops taking place on Wednesday, April 27.

The strength of the AAS annual conference is that it brings together multiple sectors focused on the common goal of preventing suicide and saving lives. Our primary objectives of AAS22 are to:

- Better equip those on the front line of prevention through the translation and application of research;
- Identify new and evolving research that will help prevent suicides;
- Embrace and integrate equity into the conference conversations;
- Integrate the voices of lived experience—including impacted family members—throughout all disciplines.

The common thread we are weaving throughout sessions and discussions is how we can continue to Widen the Lens of Suicide Prevention and be inclusive and centered on diverse experiences and perspectives. We welcome emerging, innovative areas of thought, where colleagues share developing ideas and seek collaboration to incubate and advance new approaches for effective suicide prevention.

AAS22 is an exceptional opportunity for researchers, clinicians, students, public health professionals, crisis services providers, marginalized populations, impacted families, and individuals with lived experience of loss and attempts to join together and share best practices and ideas in multiple formats. The abstract review committee will give attention to proposals approaching suicide prevention from a holistic and collaborative perspective as well as exploring the historic implementation of 988—a project that will impact the nation.

We invite you to submit proposals in one of the following formats: ① individual papers, ② posters, ③ workshops, and ④ panel discussion.

The deadline for submissions is November 12, 2021, at 11:59 p.m. EST. Unfortunately, we are not able to review late submissions, and there will not be a submission extension. Feel free to contact us or the AAS Central Office at AAS22@suicidology.org with any questions regarding this Call for Abstracts.

BEFORE YOU BEGIN YOUR ONLINE SUBMISSION

- AAS is using a new abstract management system to integrate with the new AAS database.
- In order to submit an abstract or be included as a co-author ALL presenters and co-authors/co-presenters must have a profile, including a bio, set up in the AAS database.
- You are encouraged to attend to this requirement as soon as possible. It is the responsibility of each author and co-author to create a profile and bio.
- DO NOT submit your abstract until all co-authors have been added, as you will not be able to add them afterwards.

SUBMISSION REQUIREMENTS

(1) Conference workshop abstracts should include:

- Summary of key skills, knowledge, and content to be covered;
- Description of training materials to be used, if applicable (in as much detail as possible);
- An explicit statement of the role of each presenter.

Note: Learning Objectives—two to three required within Learning Objectives Tab.

(2) Paper and poster abstracts should include:

- Research aims;
- Methods;
- Results;
- Conclusions;
- What the work adds to knowledge on the topic.

Note: Learning Objective—one required within Learning Objectives Tab.

(3) Panel abstracts should include:

- Clear description of the central issue(s) to be addressed to be included in the abstract;
- List of presenters and affiliations (no fewer than 3 and no more than 4);
- Summary of the perspective taken by each panel presenter to be included in the abstract;
- What the work adds to knowledge on the topic.

Note: Learning Objectives—two to three required within Learning Objectives Tab.

We look forward to receiving your submissions and seeing you in Chicago!

Regards,

James Charles

AAS22 Conference Chair

AAS22 Conference Planning Committee

尊敬的学界学者们：

我们很高兴地宣布，AAS22——第 55 届美国心理健康研究学会即将开始征稿！此次活动以混合形式组织，参会者可以选择出席动态的面对面会议或参加线上虚拟会议。AAS22 将于 2022 年 4 月 28 日至 30 日在芝加哥奥黑尔凯悦酒店举行，同时也在线上进行，并将于 4 月 27 日（周三）举行会前研讨会。

AAS 年会的优势在于，它将多个部门聚集在一起，专注于预防自杀和挽救生命的共同目标。AAS22 的主要目标是：

- 通过研究成果的转化和应用，更好地装备在预防第一线的人员；
- 确定有助于预防自杀的新的和不断发展的研究；
- 拥抱公平并将其纳入会议对话；

- 整合亲身经历的声音——包括受影响的家庭成员——贯穿所有的学科（专业领域）。

我们在整个会议和讨论中织就的共同主线是，我们如何继续拓宽预防自杀的视角，并以不同的经验和观点为中心。我们欢迎新兴的、创新的思想领域，在这里，同行们分享发展中的想法并寻求合作，以孵化和推进有效预防自杀的新方法。

AAS22 为研究人员、临床医生、学生、公共卫生专业人员、危机服务提供者、边缘化人群、受影响的家庭以及亲身经历过失去亲人的个人提供了一个难得的机会，并试图联合起来，以多种形式分享最佳实践和想法。摘要审查委员会将从整体和合作的角度关注自杀预防的提案，并探索 988——这一将影响国家的项目的历史性实施。

我们邀请您以以下形式之一提交提案：①个人论文；②海报；③研讨会和④小组讨论。

提交截止日期为美国东部时间 2021 年 11 月 12 日晚上 11:59。遗憾的是，我们无法审查逾期提交的内容，也不会延长提交时间。如有任何关于本次摘要征集的问题，请随时与我们或 AAS 中心办公室联系（邮箱：AAS22@suicidology.org）。

在您开始在线提交之前

- AAS 采用一种新的摘要管理系统与新的 AAS 数据库进行集成。
- 为了提交摘要或被收录为共同作者，所有发言人和共同作者 / 共同发言人必须在 AAS 数据库中建立个人资料，包括个人简介。
- 我们鼓励您尽快完成这一要求。每个作者和共同作者都有责任创建个人资料和简介。
- 在添加完所有共同作者信息之后再提交摘要，否则将无法添加。

投稿要求

（1）会议研讨会摘要应包括：

- 论文涉及的关键技能、知识和内容概述；
- 使用的培训材料说明（如适用，尽可能详细）；
- 明确说明每个发言人的角色。

注意：学习目标选项卡中需要 2～3 个学习目标。

（2）论文和海报摘要应包括：

- 研究目的；
- 研究方法；
- 研究结果；

- 结论；
- 这项工作增加了关于这个主题的什么知识。

注意：学习目标选项卡中需要列举一个学习目标。

（3）小组讨论摘要应包括：

- 摘要中要明确描述要解决的中心问题；
- 发言人及所属机构名单（不少于 3 个，不多于 4 个）；
- 摘要中包含每个小组发言人的观点概述；
- 这项工作增加了关于这个主题的什么知识。

注意：学习目标选项卡中需要列举 2～3 个学习目标。

我们期待收到您的投稿，期待在芝加哥与您见面！

顺致敬意，

詹姆斯·查尔斯

AAS22 会议主席

AAS22 会议策划委员会

12.3 会议申请（Application for Conference）

12.3.1 撰写摘要（Abstract Writing）

1. 内容和要求

申请参加国际学术会议，申请者通常不需要直接向组委会发送论文全文，而是以投稿摘要为主，不同的会务组对摘要投稿有不同的个性化要求，但总体上，摘要应包含以下要素：论文题目、研究背景与目的、研究方法、研究结果、研究结论。

下面以美国老年医学会（the Gerontological Society of America，GSA）第 71 届年会对投稿摘要的要求为例，了解会议摘要包含的要素及写作标准：

（1）Title（论文题目）

Limited to 100 characters (including spaces) and must be in title case format. Review the APA style guidelines before finalizing your title.

限制为 100 个字符（包括空格），并且必须采用标题大小写格式。在最终确定标题之前，请查看 APA 格式指南。

（2）Objectives（参会目标）

Two specific and measurable objectives are required and a third objective is optional (50 words maximum for each objective). For example, "After attending this session, participants will be able to...". Use of active verbs, such as "define" "summarize" "demonstrate", et cetera; constitute meaningful objectives.

两个具体且可衡量的目标是必需的，第三个目标是可选的（每个目标最多 50 个单词）。例如，"本次会议后，参与者将能够……"。使用主动动词，如"定义""总结""演示"等，构成有意义的目标。

（3）Abstract Body（摘要主体）

All abstracts should be unstructured with no headings, tables, or figures.

所有的摘要都应该是非结构化的，没有标题、表格或图表。

Paper and poster abstracts: maximum 250 words.

论文和海报摘要：最多 250 词。

The abstract body should include: background, methods, results, and conclusions.

摘要主体应包括：背景、方法、结果和结论。

（4）Criteria（标准）

Abstracts must be based on original scholarship. Both empirical and theoretical/conceptual contributions are welcome. Abstracts must report realized results (not anticipated results) or educational activities and/or summarize major conclusions. The following items will be considered during the review process:

摘要必须以原创学术研究为基础，欢迎实证性和理论性 / 概念性的研究成果。摘要必须报告已实现的研究结果（不是预期的结果）或教育活动和 / 或总结主要结论。在审查过程中，将考虑以下项目：

Clear statement of research aims, scholarship, or educational objectives and the significance of this work;

明确陈述研究目的、学术成就或教育目标以及本研究工作的重要性；

Specificity and appropriateness of methods;

研究方法的特异性和适当性；

Specificity of key findings (results and/or major conclusions);

关键发现（结果和 / 或主要结论）的特异性；

Clarity of implications for theory, further research, education, or practice. GSA is committed to the Reframing Aging project. Within your submission, avoid categorical terms for older adults such as "the aged" or "the elderly".

明确理论、进一步研究、教育或实践的含义。美国老年医学会致力于重构老龄化项目，在您的提交中，请避免使用诸如"the aged"或"the elderly"之类的针对老年人的绝对术语。

2. 示例

下面以编者向美国老年医学会第 71 届年会投稿的摘要进行示例展示。

The Role of Resilience and Support in the Relationship Between Loneliness and Suicide Among Nursing Home Residents

Program Area: Health Sciences

Session Code 1: Long-Term Care

Session Code 2: Mental Health

Abstract

Loneliness has been identified as a risk factor for suicidal ideation. Resilience and social support have been regarded as underlying protective factors. However, little is known about the role of resilience and social support in the relationship between loneliness and suicidal ideation among nursing home residents in China.

The purposes of this study were to investigate ① the mediating effect of resilience (as an internal resource) in the relationship between loneliness and suicidal ideation, and ② the moderating effect of social support from family, friends, and nursing staff (as external resources) in the direct or indirect effect of the mediation model.

The sample was 538 residents aged 60 or above from 37 nursing homes in Jinan, China. A moderated mediation model was conducted to explore the relationships among loneliness, resilience, social support, and suicidal ideation, after controlling for sociodemographic characteristics, physical function, cognition, and depressive symptoms.

Approximately 15% of residents (80 out of 538) were reported currently to have suicidal ideation. As expected, loneliness was positively related to suicidal ideation, while resilience and social support were negatively related to suicidal ideation. The association between loneliness and suicidal ideation was partially mediated by resilience (indirect effect 0.066, $P < 0.05$). Moreover, social support from family and nursing home staff moderated the indirect effect of loneliness on suicidal ideation through the path loneliness-resilience-suicidal ideation ($\beta = -0.111$ and $\beta = 0.212$ respectively, $P < 0.05$). Suicidal ideation is common among nursing home residents in China. Our findings underscore the important role of resilience and social support to buffer against suicidal ideation.

Learning Objective 1: After attending this session, participants will be able to define the influence of loneliness on nursing home residents' suicidal ideation.

Learning Objective 2: After attending this session, participants will be able to define the influence of resilience on nursing home residents' suicidal ideation.

Learning Objective 3: After attending this session, participants will be able to define the influence of social support on nursing home residents' suicidal ideation.

心理韧性与支持在养老院老年人孤独与自杀关系中的作用

项目领域：健康科学

会议代码 1：长期护理

会议代码 2：心理健康

摘要

孤独已被确定为自杀意念的危险因素。心理韧性和社会支持被认为是潜在的保护因素。然而，在中国养老院的老年人中，心理韧性和社会支持在孤独与自杀意念之间的关系中所起的作用尚不清楚。

本研究的目的是：①探讨心理韧性（作为内部资源）在孤独与自杀意念关系中的中介作用；②探讨家庭、朋友和护理人员的社会支持（作为外部资源）在中介模型的直接或间接效应中的调节作用。

样本是来自中国济南市 37 家养老院的 538 名 60 岁及以上的老年人。在控制社会人口学特征、身体机能、认知和抑郁症状后，采用有调节的中介模型探讨孤独感、心理韧性、社会支持和自杀意念之间的关系。

约 15% 的老年人（538 人中有 80 人）报告目前有自杀意念。正如预期的那样，孤独感与自杀意念呈正相关，而心理韧性和社会支持与自杀意念呈负相关。孤独感对自杀意念的影响受心理韧性的部分中介作用（间接效应为 0.066，$P < 0.05$）。此外，家庭和养老院工作人员的社会支持通过孤独 – 心理韧性 – 自杀意念的路径调节孤独对自杀意念的间接影响（$\beta = -0.111$ 和 $\beta = 0.212$，$P < 0.05$）。自杀意念在中国的养老院老年人中很常见。我们的研究结果强调了心理韧性和社会支持在缓冲自杀意念方面的重要作用。

学习目标 1：本次会议后，参与者将能够定义孤独对养老院老年人自杀意念的影响。

学习目标 2：本次会议后，参与者将能够定义心理韧性对养老院老年人自杀意念的影响。

学习目标 3：本次会议后，参与者将能够定义社会支持对养老院老年人自杀意念的影响。

12.3.2 邮件交流（Email Communicating）

英文邮件的写作与注意事项等内容详见本书第 2 章，本章节主要针对参加国际学术会议涉及的邮件交流进行介绍。

1. 会议邀请

在国际会议召开前，有的会议主办方会向该领域的著名学者和专家发出邀请函，邀请他们作为主题演讲嘉宾出席会议；也有的会议主办方会如本章第 2 节“会议通知”所讲的那样，在网上公开发布会议通知，然后在申请者中进行筛选，向被选中的作者发出参会邀请。这些邀请函都是正式的信函，因此应该包含所有有关参会的必要信息，并表达主办方对参加者的真诚与好客。

下面以编者收到的美国心理健康研究学会第 53 届年会的邀请函为例，学习国际学术会议邀请函的内容。

February 18, 2022

Dear Li Hua:

This letter is to invite you to present at the American Association of Mental Health's 53rd Annual Conference: “Crossroads: Preventing Suicide and Building Lives Worth Living” in Portland, Oregon, U.S. The conference will be held at the Portland Marriott Downtown Waterfront in Portland, O.R., U.S. on April 20, 2022 to April 26, 2022. Your oral presentation of “The Role of Resilience and Social Support in the Relationship Between Loneliness and Suicidal Ideation Among Chinese Nursing Home Residents” will be on Sunday April 24, 2022 at 10:45 a.m.

This conference provides a forum for those who share an interest in suicidology including physicians, researchers, psychologists, clinicians, public policy makers, and many more to share information about suicide, suicidal persons, and the repercussions of suicide. The Annual Conference is designed to meet the diverse needs of attendees while creating a powerful opportunity for networking, learning, and moving the field of suicidology forward.

Please note that this letter does not imply a commitment from the Association to provide financial support for conference registration fees, hotel fees, or travel fees. The attendee is responsible for their conference registration and for booking their own travel and lodging arrangements.

We look forward to seeing you in Portland!

Sincerely,

James Charles

Chief Executive Director

2022 年 2 月 18 日

尊敬的李华：

这封信是邀请您出席在美国俄勒冈州波特兰市举行的美国心理健康研究学会第 53 届年会："十字路口：预防自杀和构建有价值的生活"。会议将于 2022 年 4 月 20 日—4 月 26 日在美国俄勒冈州波特兰市的波特兰市中心万豪滨水酒店举行。您将于 2022 年 4 月 24 日（周日）上午 10:45 作"中国养老院老年人的孤独感和自杀意念的关系：心理韧性和社会支持的作用"的口头报告。

这次会议为那些对自杀学感兴趣的人提供了一个论坛，包括医生、研究人员、心理学家、临床医生、公共政策制定者等，以分享有关自杀、自杀者和自杀影响的信息。年会旨在满足与会者的多样化需求，同时为网络、学习和推动自杀学领域向前发展创造一个强大的机会。

请注意，这封信并不意味着协会承诺为会议注册费、住宿费或差旅费提供财务支持。与会者负责他们的会议注册以及预订自己的旅行和住宿安排。

我们期待在波特兰见到您！

谨上，

詹姆斯·查尔斯

首席执行董事

2. 接受或拒绝会议邀请的邮件通知

当你收到主办方的会议邀请并决定出席会议时，应该尽早回复邮件，通知会议主办方你已收到邀请并决定出席会议。如果你因为这样或那样的原因不能接受邀请，你也应该及时写信通知会议主办方，提前谢绝，以便让主办方有充足的时间寻找其他参会者。

1）接受邀请的回信格式

（1）Letterhead: the address of the writer 信头：作者地址

（2）Date of writing 写作日期

（3）Inside address: the address of the recipient (the conference host) 信内地址：收件人（会议主办方）的地址

（4）Salutation 称呼、称谓

（5）Body of the letter 信体

- Expressing your pleasure and honor at being invited 表达你对被邀请的荣幸
- Agreeing to do what was asked 告知你同意参会
- Repeating the main content, date, time, venue 重复邀请函中的主要内容、日期、时间、地点
- Closing the letter with your thanks, good wishes, etc. 结尾表达感谢和良好的祝愿等。

（6）Complimentary close 结束敬语

（7）Signature 签名、署名

2）谢绝邀请的回信格式

（1）Letterhead: the address of the writer 信头：作者地址

（2）Date of writing 写作日期

（3）Inside address: the address of the recipient (the conference host) 信内地址：收件人（会议主办方）的地址

（4）Salutation 称呼、称谓

（5）Body of the letter 信体

- Expressing thanks 表达感谢
- Convincing reason(s) for your refusal 令人信服的拒绝理由
- Expressing your regrets 表达你的遗憾
- Extending good wishes 致以良好祝愿

（6）Complimentary close 结束敬语

（7）Signature 签名、署名

3）示例

【例 1】

Letter of Acceptance

(Li Hua's address)

September 14, 2019

Dear Professor James Charles,

Thank you for your letter of September 13, 2019, inviting me to attend the Gerontological Society of America (GSA)'s 71st Annual Scientific Meeting to be held in Austin, Texas, the United States, November 13–17, 2019.

I am pleased to accept the invitation and will send my paper entitled "Family Care for Older Adults with Physical Dysfunction" to the Paper Committee before the required date. Thank you again for your kind invitation and I look forward to meeting you in Austin.

Sincerely yours,

(signature)

Li Hua

接受函

（李华的地址）

2019 年 9 月 14 日

尊敬的詹姆斯·查尔斯教授：

感谢您 2019 年 9 月 13 日的来信，邀请我参加将于 2019 年 11 月 13 日—17 日在美国得克萨斯州奥斯汀举行的美国老年学会第 71 届年度科学会议。

我很高兴接受邀请，并将在规定日期前将题为《躯体功能障碍老年人的家庭护理》的论文发送给论文委员会。再次感谢您的盛情邀请，期待在奥斯汀与您见面。

敬上

（签名）

李华

【例 2】

Letter of Refusal

(Li Hua's address)

May 5, 2018

Dear Professor James Charles,

Thank you for your letter of May 4, 2018, inviting me to attend the International Conference on Nursing to be held at State University of New York at Buffalo, October 6–9, 2018, as a part of the UB Centennial Celebration Conferences.

I am very sorry to inform you that I shall not be able to honor the invitation because I have been suffering from ill health for some time. I am firmly advised that it would be unwise to undertake any distance travel by air in the near future.

I wish the conference a successful one.

Respectfully yours,

(signature)

Li Hua

拒绝信

（李华的地址）

2018 年 5 月 5 日

亲爱的詹姆斯·查尔斯教授：

感谢您 2018 年 5 月 4 日的来信，邀请我参加将于 2018 年 10 月 6 日—9

日在纽约州立大学布法罗分校举行的国际护理会议，作为 UB 百年庆典会议的一部分。

我很遗憾地告知您，由于一段时间以来身体欠佳，我将无法履行邀请。医生强烈地告诫我，在不久的将来乘飞机进行任何长途旅行都是不明智的。

预祝会议取得圆满成功！

敬上

（签名）

李华

12.4 会议发言（Conference Speech）

会议发言，或称口头报告，在国际学术交流中是必不可少的。一场成功的演讲通常是精心准备和正确运用技巧的结合。尽管很难，但通过不断练习，大多数演讲者仍然可以掌握基本的技巧，从而成为学术演讲的专家。

12.4.1 撰写演讲稿（Speech Writing）

1. 内容和要求

演讲稿通常由三部分组成：引言、正文和结尾。一场成功的演讲开门见山，一开始就能抓住观众的注意力，用适当的证据说服他们，用有力的结尾给他们留下深刻的印象。

2. 常用表达

下面分别列举一些在引言、正文和结尾中常常使用的表达方式。

1）引言

学术报告的引言一般包括对主持人介绍的感谢、对观众的致意、背景介绍、报告的主题和大纲、演讲的目的等内容。演讲者可根据演讲的具体情况和讲话风格进行删减或增加。常见的引言有以下几种方式：

（1）开门见山地切入主题。例如：

- Mr. Chairman, ladies and gentlemen, the title of my presentation is... I'd like to divide my presentation into three parts. First, ...

  主席先生、女士们、先生们，我今天演讲的题目是……我想把我的演讲分成三个部分。首先，……

- Mr. Chairman, fellow colleagues, first of all, I'd like to briefly introduce the background of my paper, and then present my three points.

主席先生、各位同事，首先，我想简单介绍一下我论文的背景，然后提出我的三个观点。

- I wish to discuss... First, I will discuss... Then, I will evaluate... and suggest ways to... At last, I will conclude by...

  我想讨论……首先，我将讨论……然后，我将评价……并建议如何……最后，我将以……结束。

- Mr. Chairman, honorable guests, I'm very glad to have the opportunity to report my research on such an occasion. I'll mainly talk about three aspects. The first aspect is...

  主席先生、各位来宾，我很高兴有机会在这样的场合报告我的研究。我主要讲三个方面。第一个方面是……

- Good morning, what I am going to talk about is... First of all, I'll brief you on the terms involved in my research.

  早上好，我要讲的是……首先，我将向你们简要介绍我研究中涉及的术语。

- Good morning, ladies and gentlemen! I'm greatly enlightened by the previous speeches I have heard here. And now, I'd like to talk about my own research in three parts.

  女士们、先生们，大家早上好！我之前在这里听到的演讲给了我很大的启发。现在，我想分三个部分谈谈我自己的研究。

（2）另一种介绍演讲的方式是赞扬其他演讲者的演讲，并对自己的演讲表示出谦逊的态度。例如：

- Thank you for the warm introduction. I doubt if I can live up to that, but I'll try. Today I will talk about...

  谢谢您的热情介绍。我怀疑我是否能做到这一点，但我会努力的。今天，我将谈谈……

- OK, I greatly appreciate the opportunity to speak to you today. It's slightly improper to be talking about this topic today, but hopefully you will stay for at least part of this session and hopefully the whole session, actually. So, we've been given the task of discussing very briefly...

  好的，我非常感谢今天有机会在这里演讲。今天讨论这个话题有点不合适，但希望你们至少能听一部分，最好是整场都能听下来。因此，我们的任务是简单地讨论……

- Thank you very much. It's indeed a great pleasure to be here. It's a little bit hard to get focused on what I have to talk about after all the interesting things I've heard, particularly the last talk. I'm sitting there, thinking to myself: "Oh, my god, how I gotta explain it. It's actually a cool problem. Anyway, I'd like to tell you a little bit about what is, I have to say, a personal perspective on... As mentioned, I've been involved in this research for a long time and am doing things pretty like everybody else does. In the last one year or two, I've been rethinking about my perspectives. So, in the context of this symposium, I'd like to give you a sense of what that is all about."

非常感谢，很高兴来到这里。在我听了那么多有趣的演讲，特别是在上一场演讲之后，我很难集中注意力在我要讲的内容上。我坐在那里，对自己说："天哪，我该怎么解释。这实际上是一个很酷的问题。无论如何，我想告诉你们一点，我个人对于……的观点。如前所述，我已经参与这项研究很长时间了，我做的事情和其他人一样。在过去的一两年里，我一直在反思我的观点。所以，在这次研讨会的背景下，我想让你们对这一切有个大概的了解。"

（3）对大会主席及组委会表示感谢。通常，在演讲者上台之前，主席会简短地介绍演讲者。因此，在演讲开始时，演讲者应首先对主席表示感谢，并对能与来自同一专业领域的专家会面感到激动。例如：

- Mr. Chairman! Ladies and gentlemen! I am greatly honored to be invited to address this conference.

  主席先生！女士们、先生们！我非常荣幸被邀请在这次会议上发言。

- Mr. Chairman, first let me express my gratitude to you and your staff for allowing me to participate in this very exciting meeting.

  主席先生，首先请允许我向您和您的工作人员表示感谢，感谢你们允许我参加这次激动人心的会议。

- Thank you, Mr. Chairman, for your very kind introduction. Mr. Chairman, ladies and gentlemen, I consider it a great honor to be asked to speak about... on this session.

  谢谢主席先生，感谢您的亲切介绍。主席先生、女士们、先生们，我很荣幸被邀请在这届会议上谈论……

- Good morning, it is a great honor for me to be here with you this morning and to share my ideas with such distinguished colleagues. I want to thank... and... for their hard work in holding this conference. I want to especially thank Dr. ..., the Director of the Center. My thanks to him are much broader than for this conference, though. ... has been a mentor to me, as he has too many others in... and beyond, and I believe that all of us have been enriched by his generosity.

早上好，我很荣幸能在这里与各位杰出的同事们分享我的想法。我要感谢……和……为举办这次会议所做的辛勤工作。我要特别感谢中心主任……博士，不过我对他的感谢比对这次会议的感谢要广泛得多。……一直是我的导师，就像他对……内外的许多人一样，我相信我们所有人都因他的慷慨而受益匪浅。

- Good morning, ladies and gentlemen. It's a great honor and pleasure to speak to you this morning. Congratulations, ..., director of the ... Association, for putting this conference together. And thank you ..., for your good work and wonderful comments. I want to begin by thanking everyone in this room for the important work you are doing. Today, I want to talk to you about... Let me begin by...

  女士们、先生们，大家早上好。今天早上和你们讲话是我莫大的荣幸。祝贺……协会主任……，组织这次会议。谢谢……的出色工作和精彩评论。首先，我要感谢在座的每一位，感谢你们所做的重要工作。今天，我想和大家谈谈……让我先从……

- Thank you, Mr. Chairman. Ladies and gentlemen, I appreciate the opportunity to be with you today. I am here to talk to you about...

  谢谢主席先生。女士们、先生们，我很高兴今天有机会和大家一起。我来这里是想跟大家谈谈……

- Dear colleagues, first of all, I would like to thank Mr. Chairman and our generous hosts for providing me with such a precious opportunity to meet, exchange views, and share thoughts with so many experts and scholars in my field. What I would like to talk about is...

  尊敬的各位同行，首先，我要感谢主席先生和慷慨的东道主为我提供这样一个宝贵的机会，与这么多我所在领域的专家学者会面、交换意见、分享想法。我想说的是……

- Mr. Chairman, thank you for your warm introduction and also for your efforts in making the opening of this medical conference so successful. Now I would like to say something about my study...

  主席先生，感谢您的热情介绍，也感谢您为这次医学会议的成功开幕所做的努力。现在，我想谈谈我的研究……

- Thank you, Mr. Chairman, Mr. Director-General, distinguished members of... and friends, good morning, it's a great honor to be here today...

  谢谢主席先生、总干事先生、尊敬的……委员和朋友们，早上好，今天很荣幸来到这里……

（4）以机智幽默的语言介绍。学术会议通常是严肃的，在一系列的讲座和讨论之后，参与者可能会感到疲惫。在这种情况下，演讲者可能会用幽默或机智的介绍来娱乐观众，改变会议的严肃气氛。例如：

- Mr. Chairman, ladies and gentlemen, there is a Chinese saying "with a hare under one's garment" to describe the uneasiness of a nervous person. That is how I am feeling at such a moment, and before such a big audience, there seems to be a hare under my garment. Well, now, speaking about nervousness, I would like to show you the result of my experiment on the nervous system of a rabbit...

  主席先生，女士们、先生们，中国有句俗语"衣兜里藏着一只兔子"来形容一个人的紧张不安。这就是我此刻的感受，在这么多观众面前，我的衣服里好像藏着一只兔子。好吧，现在，说到紧张，我想向你们展示一下我对兔子神经系统的实验结果……

（5）即兴介绍。有时，由于情况的意外变化，准备好的开场引言可能显得不合适或不充分。在这种情况下，有经验的演讲者可能会根据情况即兴开场，这也许会引起观众的兴趣。例如：

- In his paper, Dr. ... has presented an admirably clear and concise account of the... I would, however, like to call your attention to an aspect of the...

  在他的论文中，……博士对……给出了令人钦佩的清晰而简洁的描述。然而，我想提请你们注意……的一个方面。

- I can see many of you are from... department.

  我看到你们中很多人来自……部门。

- I understand that after long hours of discussion sessions, you must feel a little tired. Now I'd like you to see an interesting topic.

  我知道经过长时间的讨论，你们一定感到有点累了。现在，我想让你们看一个有趣的话题。

（6）道歉式引言。如果演讲者认为观众很难理解他 / 她要说的话，则可能会以道歉形式开始介绍。例如：

- Good morning, ladies and gentlemen. I must apologize for speaking somewhat technically today, but I think it is difficult to talk about this theory without being a little bit technical.

  女士们、先生们，大家早上好。我必须为今天的演讲有点技术性而道歉，但我认为要谈论这个理论很难不涉及一点技术性。

2）正文

医学报告的正文是学术报告中最重要的部分，通常包括研究方法、研究目标、研究结果等。演讲时，如果观众知道演讲者讲话的结构和顺序，这对演讲的效果很有帮助。演讲时，演讲者应合理使用一些信号语言，让观众对演讲的逻辑和条理有一个整体的认识。

（1）让观众了解“我在讲什么”。例如：

- In this part of my paper, I'll inform you about...
  在我论文的这一部分，我将告诉你们关于……
- So, let me first give you a brief overview of...
  所以，让我先给你们一个简短的概述……
- What I aim to do first is to explain a few key concepts...
  我首先要做的是解释几个关键概念……
- What I would like to do now is to show you a brief introduction of the research project itself.
  我现在想做的是向你们简要介绍一下这个研究项目本身。
- What we need to do first is looking at some of the problems which we set out to solve.
  我们首先需要做的是研究一下我们需要着手解决的一些问题。

（2）让观众了解“我下面要讲什么”。例如：

- This leads me directly to the next part of my talk.
  这就把我直接引到我演讲的下一部分。
- This now brings us to my second point.
  这就引出了我的第二点。
- Let's move on to the next issue...
  让我们继续下一个问题……
- So, now I'd like to turn to my next question.
  所以，现在我想转向我的下一个问题。

（3）暗示即将结尾。例如：

- This brings me to the end of my second point.
  我的第二点到此结束。
- That's all I wanted to say about...
  这就是所有我想说的……
- So much for...
  ……到此为止。

（4）总结一个观点。例如：

- I'd now like to sum up the main points for you.
  现在，我想为大家总结一下要点。
- Let me briefly summarize what I've said so far.
  让我简单总结一下到目前为止我所讲的内容。
- Before I conclude my talk, let me go through the main issues once more.
  在结束演讲之前，让我把主要问题再过一遍。

（5）要点排序。例如：

- To begin with / At the beginning / At the start / First(ly)
  在开头 / 首先
- Then / Next / After that / Second(ly)
  然后 / 接下来 / 在那之后 / 第二
- Finally / At the end / Last(ly)
  最后

3）结尾

结尾是演讲的另一个重要部分，通常，一个令人印象深刻的结尾可以让观众更容易记住演讲要点。下面介绍几种不同类型的结尾。

（1）直截了当式结尾。这种结尾通常是一个简短的结论性陈述。例如：

- Let me just wind up here.
  我就在这里结束吧。
- I'll stop here. Thank you.
  我就讲到这里。谢谢你们！
- That's all. Thank you, Mr. Chairman. Thank you all.
  就这样。谢谢主席先生，谢谢大家。
- That's all I want to say at present. Thank you, ladies and gentlemen.
  这就是我目前想说的全部内容。谢谢大家，女士们、先生们。
- Well, I think this is a good place to wind up my talk. Thank you everyone for your attention!
  我想这是结束我演讲的适当时机。谢谢大家的关注！

（2）致谢式结尾。这种结尾是指在结束时向对论文提供过帮助的人表达感谢。例如：

- I'd like to, of course, thank my fellow colleagues publicly. They are the most marvelous and smart people I've ever had the privilege to work with. They are really fantastic. And it's also been a pleasure to come here. Thank you very much.

当然，我要公开感谢我的同事们，他们是我有幸共事过的最了不起、最聪明的人。他们真的很棒。我也很高兴来到这里，非常感谢。

（3）总结式结尾。用一个简洁的总结作为演讲的结尾是一种常见的方式。例如：

- Now, let me repeat this in a different form.
  现在，让我用另一种形式重复一遍。
- Now let me review what I have said so far about...
  现在，让我回顾一下到目前为止我所说的关于……
- Now let me end by emphasizing the main points once again.
  最后，让我再次强调要点。
- I would like now to summarize... which we have been talking about.
  现在，我想总结一下……这是我们一直在讨论的问题。
- In summary, ...
  简要地说 / 概括地说 / 总的来说，……
- The themes I have dealt with can be boiled down as follows: ...
  我所讨论的主题可以概括如下：……
- In case I have made any careless mistakes and in order to clarify what I have said, let me just go over the main points again... that's all. Thank you, everyone.
  如果我犯了什么粗心的错误，为了澄清我所说的，让我把要点再过一遍……就这样，谢谢大家。
- Now, I want to answer the title question, what is...?
  现在，我想回答标题中的问题，什么是……？

（4）征求意见式结尾。这是在演讲即将结束时，向观众征求意见或建议的结尾方式，这种结尾方式体现了演讲者的谦逊态度和对观众的尊重，有助于增强演讲的互动性和观众的参与感。例如：

- Now that I have finished my speech, I hope you'll give me your comments and suggestions. They'll help me improve my work.
  现在，我的演讲结束了，希望你们能给我提出你们的意见和建议，这样可以帮助我改进我的工作。
- Thank you for the opportunity to share some of the work my office has done related to... I am happy to address any questions.

感谢你们给我机会分享我们全体工作人员所做的与……有关的工作。我很乐意回答任何问题。

- That's all for my talk. If there are any points that I didn't make clearly, please point them out and I would like to give further explanation.

  我的演讲到此结束。如果有什么我没有说清楚的地方，请指出来，我愿意进一步解释。

- To conclude, it seems that if we are to succeed in solving the many interrelated problems of..., only the fullest and most intelligent use of... will enable us to do so. That's all, thank you.

  总之，如果我们要成功地解决许多与……相互关联的问题，似乎我们只有充分、明智地利用……才可以。就这样，谢谢大家。

- As time is limited, I can just give you the outline of what I've been studying. For any questions to be raised, I'm quite willing to discuss them with you at any time. Thank you.

  由于时间有限，我只能给你们简要地讲一下我所研究的内容。如果有任何问题，我很愿意随时与你们讨论。谢谢大家！

- That's all for my talk. Please don't hesitate to put forward your suggestions and advice, if you have any. Thank you.

  我的演讲到此结束。如果有什么建议和意见，请尽管提出来。谢谢！

3. 示例

【例 1】

Good morning, ladies and gentlemen. The topic of my presentation today is... The aim of my presentation is to... The main points I will be talking about are... Finally, I'll be happy to answer your questions at the end.

女士们、先生们，大家早上好。我今天演讲的主题是……我演讲的目的是……我要讲的要点是……最后，我很乐意回答大家的问题。

【例 2】

Firstly, I'd like to talk about... I'd like to illustrate this by showing you this graphic...

首先，我想谈谈……我想通过这张图来说明这个问题……

【例 3】

That's all for my first topic.

这就是我的第一个主题。

【例 4】

I'd now like to conclude by summing up and making some recommendations. The purpose of this presentation is to... The main points I have talked about are...

最后，我想总结一下并提出一些建议。这次演讲的目的是……我所谈到的主要观点是……

【例 5】

I'd now like to invite any questions you may have.

现在请大家提问。

12.4.2 幻灯片制作（Slides Producing）

1. 内容和要求

国际学术会议报告幻灯片的主要内容应围绕要报告的论文展开，主要包含以下几项：

（1）标题（大会名称、报告标题、作者姓名和单位）（Title）；

（2）目录（Contents）；

（3）研究背景（Background）；

（4）研究内容（Contents）；

（5）研究方法（Methods）；

（6）研究结果（Results）；

（7）讨论（Discussion）；

（8）局限性（Limitation）；

（9）结论（Conclusion）；

（10）致谢（Acknowledgement）；

（11）结尾（Ending）。

国际学术会议一般只对报告的时间和主旨有所要求，而不对幻灯形式提出具体要求，但优秀的学术报告幻灯片通常要做到模板和风格统一、逻辑清晰、重点突出、图表丰富、文字以关键字作为提示，避免大篇幅文字、照本宣科。

2. 示例

【例】

下面以编者在第六届齐鲁护理国际青年学者论坛（The 6th Qilu International Young Nursing Scholars Forum）所作的报告为例，展示幻灯片的制作与内容要素。

第一步，展示论坛名称以及报告的标题和作者。

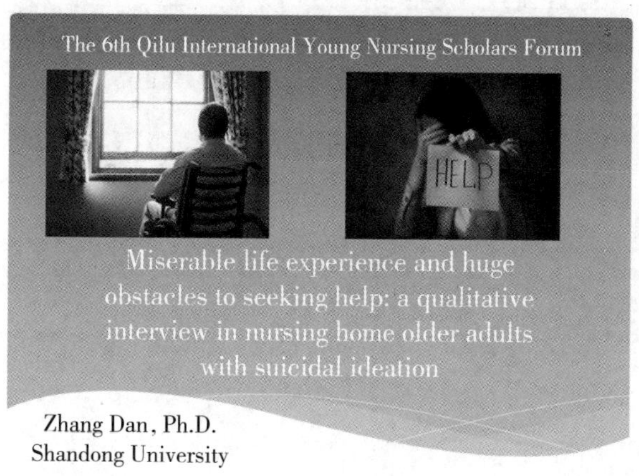
The 6th Qilu International Young Nursing Scholars Forum
HELP
Miserable life experience and huge obstacles to seeking help: a qualitative interview in nursing home older adults with suicidal ideation
Zhang Dan, Ph.D.
Shandong University

图 12.1　幻灯片封面

第二步，通过目录介绍本次报告的主要内容。

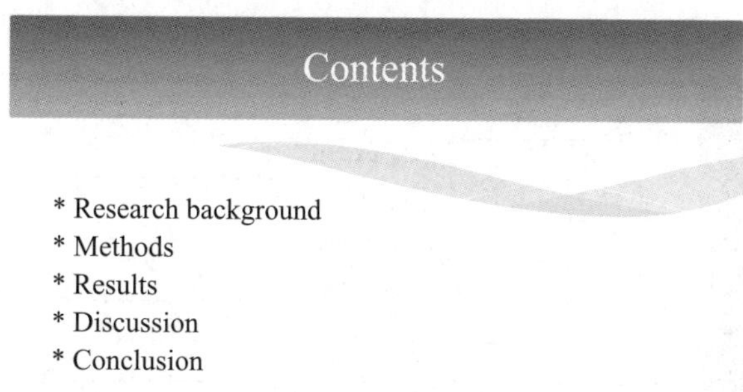

图 12.2　幻灯片目录

第三步，在正式报告每一部分的内容之前，用小标题页进行提示。

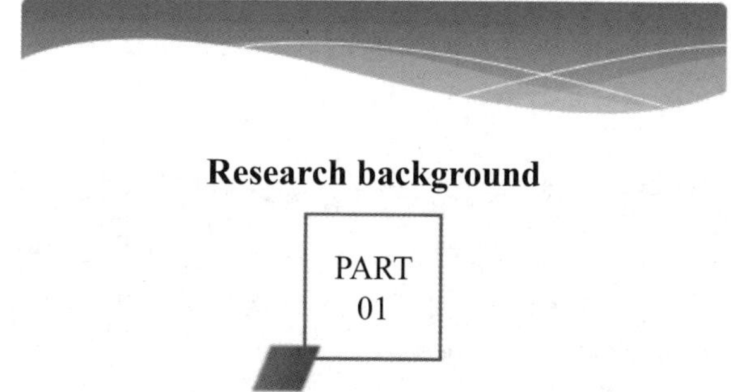

图 12.3　幻灯片小标题页

第四步，开始正式内容的报告，注意幻灯片的简洁和清晰，尤其在结果部分尽量使用图表进行展示，例如：

Findings from our previous quantitative analysis

➢ 538 older adults living in 37 nursing homes in Jinan, Shandong

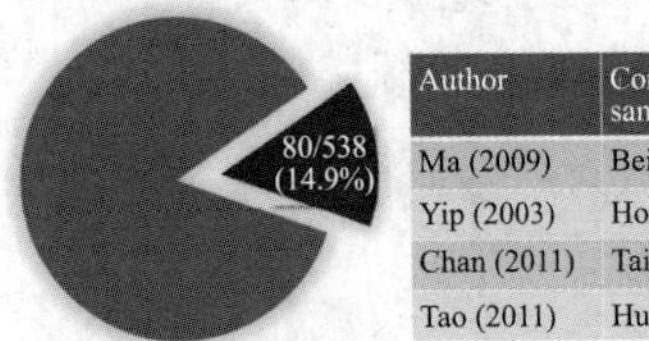

Author	Community samples	Suicide ideation (%)
Ma (2009)	Beijing (1159)	2.2
Yip (2003)	Hong Kong (917)	6.0
Chan (2011)	Taiwan (3853)	6.1
Tao (2011)	Hunan (670)	13.0

■ With suicidal ideation
■ Without suicidal ideation

9

图 12.4　幻灯片内容（饼状图和表格）

Suicide in older adults

China Health Statistical Yearbook–2020

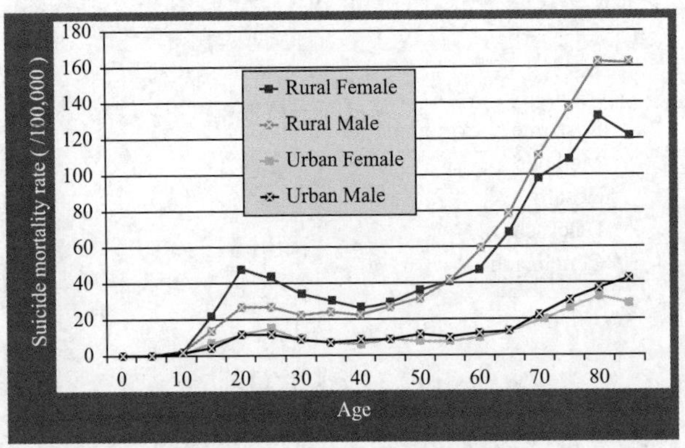

图 12.5　幻灯片内容（折线图）

最后，在报告内容展示完毕后，演讲者需要在结尾页面表达对会议主办方和观众的感谢，并留下自己的联系方式。

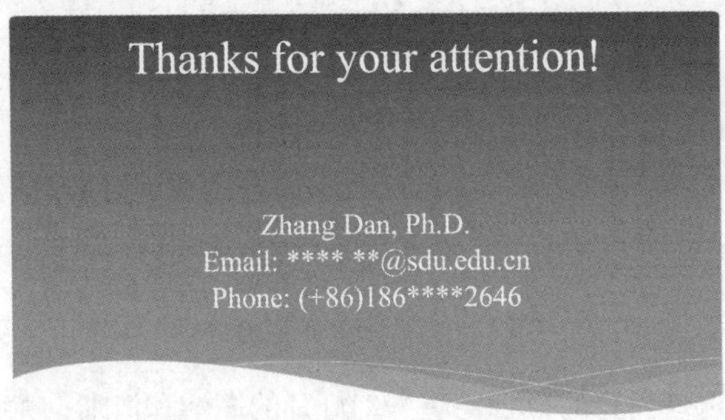
Thanks for your attention!
Zhang Dan, Ph.D.
Email: **** **@sdu.edu.cn
Phone: (+86)186****2646

图 12.6　幻灯片致谢页

Exercises

Exercise I　Translate the following conference notice into Chinese.

GSA 2022—The Gerontological Society of America (GSA) Annual Scientific Meeting

Meeting Location: Orlando, FL

Meeting Dates: Thursday, May 12–Saturday, May 14

Abstract Submission Deadline: December 1, 2021, 11:15 p.m. E.T.

Research Abstract Acceptance Email Notifications: Late February

The GSA Annual Scientific Meeting is the premier educational event in geriatrics, providing the latest information on clinical care, research on aging, and innovative models of care delivery. Held annually, the GSA Annual Scientific Meeting addresses the educational needs of geriatrics professionals from all disciplines. Physicians, nurses, pharmacists, physician assistants, social workers, long-term care and managed care providers, health care administrators, and others can update their knowledge and skills through state-of-the-art educational sessions, including invited symposia, workshops, and meet-the-expert sessions.

Abstracts are solicited in the following categories:

- Case Series & Case Studies
- Clinical Innovation & Quality Improvement
- Clinical Trials & Epidemiology
- Ethics & Qualitative Research
- Geriatric Bioscience & Geriatric Education
- Geriatric Medicine in Other Specialties
- Geriatric Syndromes
- Health Services & Policy Research
- Neurologic & Behavioral Science

Exercise II　Translate the following conference paper abstract into English.

目的：了解中青年血液系统肿瘤患者的治疗期症状群经历情况，探讨症状群的影响因素。

方法：于 2020 年 9 月至 2021 年 8 月，选取了山东省济南市两所三甲医院的 315

名中青年血液系统肿瘤患者。通过研究者自行设计的一般资料调查表、安德森症状评估量表、患者尊严量表、一般自我效能感量表和健康状况调查简表对患者进行调查。使用 SPSS21.0 软件进行研究数据的分析，分析步骤依次为：描述性分析、单因素分析、多元线性回归分析。

结果：中青年血液系统肿瘤患者的症状发生率排在前五位的依次是疲劳（乏力）（81.6%）、胃口差（74.9%）、苦恼（73.7%）、口干（73.7%）、睡眠不安（70.5%）。以症状群为因变量进行单因素分析显示，中青年患者的性别、婚姻状况、个人月收入、肿瘤类型等变量在症状群得分上的分布差异具有统计学意义（$P < 0.05$）。多元回归分析结果显示，个人月收入可单独解释症状群 19.1% 的变异（β = –0.175，R2 = 0.191），其次是性别（β = –0.133，R2 = 0.239）、肿瘤类型（β = –0.117，R2 = 0.266）。

结论：中青年血液系统肿瘤患者在治疗期会出现多种症状，其中疲劳（乏力）的发生率最高且最严重，患者的情绪症状亦较为突出，应加以重视。症状群的影响因素包括性别、婚姻状况、个人月收入、肿瘤类型。因此，未来的研究可从性别对照的角度出发，以对患者的症状管理策略提供更多的理论指导。

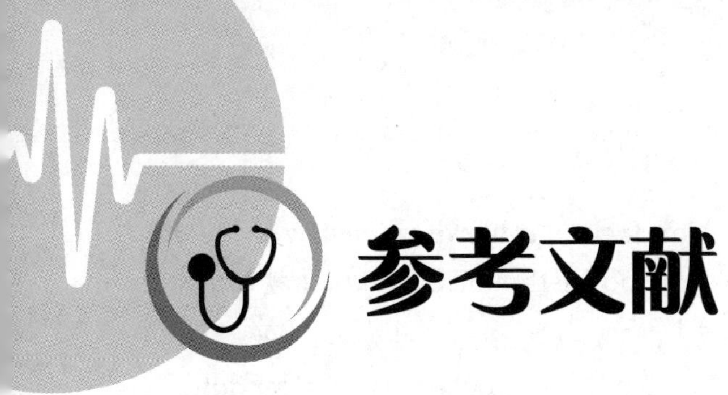

参考文献

陈晓明 . 2009. 医学论文英语摘要的结构及语言特点 . 英语知识，(8): 24–26.

国家食品药品监督管理局 . 2022. 化学药品及治疗用生物制品说明书通用格式和撰写指南 . 5 月 20 日 . 来自国家药品监督管理局药审中心 .

国家药典委员会 . 2020. 中华人民共和国药典（二部）. 北京：中国中医药科技出版社 .

何筑丽，国林祥 . 2022. 医学英语写作与翻译 . 北京：高等教育出版社 .

黄栩兵 . 2004. 第十三讲 文献综述的写作 . 人民军医，47（4）: 241–243.

李朝品，王先寅 . 2021. 医学论文英文摘要写作 . 3 版 . 北京：科技出版社 .

李传英，潘承礼 . 2014. 医学英语写作与翻译 . 武汉：武汉大学出版社 .

李根林 . 2003. 如何撰写医学文献综述 . 中华眼科杂志，(8): 61–63.

李康，等 . 2013. 医学统计学 . 北京：人民卫生出版社 .

南肇胜 . 1995. 如何撰写医学文献综述论文 . 临床医学，(3): 28–31.

潘雪，等 . 2021. 医学期刊出版伦理审查的实践与思考——以《中华内分泌外科杂志》为例 . 编辑报，33（6）: 635–638.

彭晓霞，等 . 2009. 病例报告的临床价值、科研意义与撰写规范 . 中国卒中杂志，4（3）: 259–264.

王亚娜，陈春林 . 2012. 医学伦理视角下的 SCI 生物医学英语论文 . 中国医学伦理学，25（4）: 538–541.

萧惠来 . 2020. 药物说明书撰写指南（供化学药品和治疗用生物制品用）. 北京：化学工业出版社 .

薛绍莲 . 2003. 怎样提高医学文献综述的写作水平 . 国外医学（生理、病理科学与临床分册）,（2）: 219–220.

杨树隽，薛廷民 . 2020. 英语医学论文写作教程 . 北京：人民卫生出版社 .

杨思兰，等 . 2020. 医学研究中常见的综述类型及相关方法分析 . 中华护理教育，17（2）: 179–185.

周英智，等 . 2008. 医学期刊稿约中伦理学要求现况调查 . 中国科技期刊研究，19（5）: 779–781.

Ahmed, S., Vaska, M. & Turin, T. C. 2016. Conducting a literature review in health research: Basics of the approach, typology and methodology. *Journal of National Heart Foundation of Bangladesh, 5*(2): 44–51.

Altuntas, F., Altuntas, S. & Dereli, T. 2022. Social network analysis of tourism data: A case study of quarantine decisions in COVID-19 pandemic. *International Journal of Information Management Data Insights, 2*(2): 100–108.

Alving, B. E., Christensen, J. B. & Thrysøe, L. 2018. Hospital nurses' information retrieval behaviours in relation to evidence based nursing: A literature review. *Health Information & Libraries Journal, 35*(1): 3–23.

Amass, T. et al. 2022. Stress-related disorders of family members of patients admitted to the intensive care unit with COVID-19. *JAMA Internal Medicine, 182*(6): 624–633.

Anon. 2019. Structure for writing an effective clinical review articles. *Pubrica*. Retrieved December 20, 2023, from Pubrica website.

Chai, H. et al. 2021. Hypertension is associated with osteoporosis: A case-control study in Chinese postmenopausal women. *BMC Musculoskeletal Disorders*, (22): 1–7.

Chung, M. et al. 2020. CT imaging features of 2019 novel coronavirus (2019-nCoV). *Radiology, 295*(1): 202–207.

Dowling, L. et al. 2022. A novel presentation of nasal steatocystoma simplex: A case report and literature review. *JAMA Otolaryngology—Head & Neck Surgery, 148*(4): 380–381.

Fike, C. D. & Hansen, T. N. 1989. The effect of alkalosis on hypoxia-induced pulmonary vasoconstriction in lungs of newborn rabbits. *Pediatric Research, 25*(4): 383–388.

Forero, R. et al. 2012. A literature review on care at the end-of-life in the emergency department. *Emergency Medicine International*, (2012): 486–516.

Gambescia, S. F. 2013. A brief on writing a successful abstract. *Education for Health, 26*(2): 122–125.

Grant, M. J. & Booth, A. 2009. A typology of reviews: An analysis of 14 review types and associated methodologies. *Health Information & Libraries Journal, 26*(2): 91–108.

Griffin, D. O. et al. 2020. Pulmonary embolism and increased levels of d-dimer in patients with coronavirus disease. *Emerg Infect Dis., 26*(8): 1941–1943.

Haworth, R. N. & Ball, C. S. 1981. Heat stroke in October: A case report. *BMJ Military Health, 127*(2): 82–84.

Hay, S. M., Hay, F. A. & Austwick, D. H. 1992. Case report. Bee sting brachial block. *Emergency Medicine Journal*, *9*(4): 369–372.

Ickes, M. J. & Gambescia, S. F. 2011. Abstract art: How to write competitive conference and journal abstracts. *Health Promotion Practice*, *12*(4): 493–496.

Ishi, Y. et al. 2015. Case report: Trigeminal neuralgia caused by a minute meningioma with hyperostosed suprameatal tubercle. *Case Reports in Neurology*, *7*(2): 167–172.

Jeffrey, M. N. & Jeffrey, M. J. 1987. Conjunctival amyloid—A case report. *Journal of the Royal Naval Medical Service*, *73*(2): 115–117.

Jia, P. et al. 2017. Hypertriglyceridemia and atherosclerosis. *Lipids in Health & Disease*, *16*(1): 233.

Khan, G. Q. et al. 2003. Salmonella typhi endocarditis: A case report. *Journal of Clinical Pathology*, *56*(10): 801–802.

Kokkinos, P. et al. 2008. Exercise capacity and mortality in black and white men. *Circulation*, *117*(5): 614–622.

Link-Gelles, R. et al. 2022. Public health response to a case of paralytic poliomyelitis in an unvaccinated person and detection of poliovirus in wastewater—New York, June–August 2022. *Morbidity and Mortality Weekly Report*, *71*(33): 1065.

Lucarelli, K. M., Chen, K. G. & Akella, S. S. 2022. An unusual case of severe bilateral extraocular muscle enlargement. *JAMA Ophthalmology*, *140*(7): 738–739.

Mamede, S. & Schmidt, H. G. 2017. Reflection in medical diagnosis: A literature review. *Health Professions Education*, *3*(1): 15–25.

Marckmann, P. et al. 1989. Imported pedal chancroid: Case report. *Sexually Transmitted Infections*, *65*(2): 126–127.

Merritt, C. J., De Zoysa, N. & Hutton, J. M. 2017. A qualitative study of younger men's experience of heart attack (myocardial infarction). *British Journal of Health Psychology*, *22*(3): 589–608.

Morey, M. C. 2019. Physical activity and exercise in older adults. *UpToDate, Waltham.* Retrieved April 11, 2015, from UpToDate, Waltham website.

Morin, C. M. et al. 1999. Behavioral and pharmacological therapies for late-life insomnia: A randomized controlled trial. *JAMA*, *281*(11): 991–999.

Patel, B., Ladva, Z. R. & Khan, U. 2015. Hemichorea-hemiballism: A case report. *Practical Neurology*, *15*(3): 222–223.

Peters, U., Dixon, A. E. & Forno, E. 2018. Obesity and asthma. *Journal of Allergy and Clinical Immunology*, *141*(4): 1169–1179.

Redman, L. M. et al. 2021. Attenuated early pregnancy weight gain by prenatal lifestyle interventions does not prevent gestational diabetes in the LIFE-Moms consortium. *Diabetes Research and Clinical Practice*, (171): 108–549.

Shorey, S. & Chua, C. 2022. Nurses and nursing students' experiences on pediatric end-of-life care and death: A qualitative systematic review. *Nurse Education Today*, (112): 105–332.

Shortal, B. P. et al. 2019. Duration of EEG suppression does not predict recovery time or degree of cognitive impairment after general anaesthesia in human volunteers. *British Journal of Anaesthesia*, *123*(2): 206–218.

Vanholder, R. et al. 2021. Organ donation and transplantation: A multi-stakeholder call to action. *Nature Reviews Nephrology*, *17*(8): 554–568.

Weizman, O. et al. 2022. Machine learning-based scoring system to predict in-hospital outcomes in patients hospitalized with COVID-19. *Archives of Cardiovascular Diseases*, *115*(12): 617–626.

Williams, G. & Rees, J. 2007. *100 Cases in Clinical Medicine*. Frederick: Hodder Education.

Yoon, H. Y. & Uh, S. T. 2022. Post-coronavirus disease 2019 pulmonary fibrosis: Wait or needs intervention. *Tuberculosis and Respiratory Diseases*, *85*(4): 320.

Zeiger, M. 2000. Essentials of writing biomedical research papers. *Discourse and Writing/Rédactologie*, *11*(1): 33–36.